OXFORD CARDIOLOGY LIBRARY

Chronic Heart Failure

O C L
OXFORD CARDIOLOGY LIBRARY

Chronic Heart Failure

Edited by

Professor Mark Kearney

Professor of Cardiology and Honorary
Consultant Cardiologist,
University of Leeds,
Leeds, UK

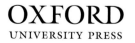

OXFORD
UNIVERSITY PRESS

OXFORD

UNIVERSITY PRESS

Great Clarendon Street, Oxford OX2 6DP

Oxford University Press is a department of the University of Oxford.
It furthers the University's objective of excellence in research, scholarship,
and education by publishing worldwide in

Oxford New York

Auckland Cape Town Dar es Salaam Hong Kong Karachi
Kuala Lumpur Madrid Melbourne Mexico City Nairobi
New Delhi Shanghai Taipei Toronto

With offices in

Argentina Austria Brazil Chile Czech Republic France Greece
Guatemala Hungary Italy Japan Poland Portugal Singapore
South Korea Switzerland Thailand Turkey Ukraine Vietnam

Oxford is a registered trade mark of Oxford University Press
in the UK and in certain other countries

Published in the United States
by Oxford University Press Inc., New York

British Library Cataloguing in Publication Data

Data available

Library of Congress Cataloging in Publication Data

Data available

Typeset by Newgen Imaging Systems (P) Ltd., Chennai, India
Printed in Italy
on acid-free paper by
Legoprint S.p.a
ISBN 978-0-19-954233-8

10 9 8 7 6 5 4 3 2 1

Whilst every effort has been made to ensure that the contents of this book are as
complete, accurate and-up-to-date as possible at the date of writing. Oxford
University Press is not able to give any guarantee or assurance that such is the case.
Readers are urged to take appropriately qualified medical advice in all cases. The
information in this book is intended to be useful to the general reader, but should
not be used as a means o self-diagnosis or for the prescription of medication.

Contents

Preface

Chronic heart failure is a major healthcare issue, which every health-care professional will encounter at some point. It is a highly complex disorder that remains a therapeutic challenge. Our understanding of the pathophysiology and management of chronic heart failure have developed at an amazing rate over the last 20 years. It seems like only yesterday that, as a house officer, I was admitting patients to hospital to commence an angiotensin-converting-enzyme inhibitor. Moreover, if you had suggested at that time that patients with heart failure should receive a beta-blocker you would have been laughed at. As the population ages more and more people are suffering from chronic heart failure. Their outlook is now substantially better than it was when I was a house officer. Patients can be offered life-prolonging drugs, devices, and surgery. It may be that in another 20 years heart failure will not be the malignant disease it is considered to be now.

I am indebted to all the contributors to this book for their support, enthusiasm, and willingness to share their expertise. Chronic heart failure is such a complex disorder that it is inevitable that there will be some areas that readers may feel I have neglected or overemphasised. That is entirely my fault. However, I believe that this book draws on the expertise on a range of leaders in their field and I hope that readers enjoy reading their work as much as I did.

Mark Kearney
November 2007

Contributors

Dr Khaled Abouani
Research Fellow in Cardiology,
Cardiothoracic Centre,
Liverpool, UK

Dr Dirk Brutsaert
Centre of Heart Failure and
Cardiac Rehabilitation,
University of Antwerp,
Belgium

Dr Richard Cubbon
British Heart Foundation
Research Fellow,
Division of Cardiovascular
and Diabetes Research,
University of Leeds, UK

Dr Edward Duncan
British Heart Foundation
Research Fellow and
Registrar in Cardiology,
King's College London, UK

Dr Carey Edwards
Research Fellow in Cardiology,
King's College Hospital,
London, UK

Dr Christopher Gale
Clinical Lecturer in Cardiology,
Division of Cardiovascular and
Diabetes Research,
University of Leeds, UK

Marc Goethals
Consultant Cardiologist,
Cardiovascular Centre,
OLV Hospital,
Aalst, Belgium

Dr Alan Japp
British Heart Foundation
Research Fellow and Registrar
in Cardiology,
University of Edinburgh, UK

Prof. Mark Kearney
Professor of Cardiology and
Consultant Cardiologist,
Division of Cardiovascular and
Diabetes Research,
University of Leeds, UK

Dr Gilles W. De Keulenaer
Centre of Heart Failure and
Cardiac Rehabilitation,
University of Antwerp,
Belgium

Dr Ninian Lang
British Heart Foundation
Research Fellow and Registrar
in Cardiology,
University of Edinburgh, UK

Dr Nigel Lewis
British Heart Foundation
Research Fellow,
Division of Cardiovascular
and Diabetes Research,
University of Leeds, UK

John MacDonald
Cardiology Registrar,
Manchester Royal
Infirmary, UK

Dr Narbeh Melikian
Clinical Lecturer in Cardiology,
King's College London, UK

CONTRIBUTORS

Prof. David Newby
Professor of Cardiology and
Consultant Cardiologist,
University of Edinburgh, UK

Dr Robin Ray
British Heart Foundation
Research Fellow and Registrar
in Cardiology,
King's College London, UK

Prof. Ajay Shah
British Heart Foundation
Professor of Cardiology and
Consultant Cardiologist,
King's College London, UK

Dr Sanjay Sharma
Consultant Cardiologist,
King's College Hospital,
London, UK

Stephen Shaw
Cardiology Registrar,
Manchester Royal Infirmary, UK

Dr Iain Squire
Senior Lecturer in Cardiology,
University of Leicester, UK

Prof. Lip-Bun Tan
Professor of Cardiovascular
Medicine,
Division of Cardiovascular and
Diabetes Research,
University of Leeds, UK

Dr Mark Vanderheyden
Consultant Cardiologist,
Cardiovascular Centre,
OLV Hospital,
Aalst, Belgium

Simon Williams
Consultant Cardiologist,
Manchester Royal Infirmary, UK

Dr David Justin Wright
Consultant Cardiologist,
Cardiothoracic Centre,
Liverpool, UK

Abbreviations

ACE	angiotensin-converting enzyme
ACEI	angiotensin-converting enzyme inhibitor
ACTH	adrenocorticotrophin
ADH	anti-diuretic hormone
ARVC	arrhythmogenic right-ventricular cardiomyopathy
BNP	brain natriuretic peptide
CABG	coronary artery bypass surgery
CARE-HF	Cardiac Resynchronization in Heart Failure study
CIBIS	Cardiac Insufficiency Bisoprolol Study
CHARM	Candesartan in Heart Failure Assessment of Reduction in Mortality and Morbidity trial
CHF	chronic heart failure
CKD	chronic kidney disease
CMR	cardiac magnetic resonance (imaging)
COMET	Carvedilol or Metoprolol European Trial
COMPANION	Comparison of Medical Therapy Pacing and Defibrillation in Heart Failure
CONSENSUS	Cooperative North Scandinavian Enalapril Survival Study
COPD	chronic obstructive pulmonary disease
COPERNICUS	The Effect of Carvedilol on Survival in Severe Chronic Heart Failure trial
CPAP	continuous positive airways pressure
CRT	cardiac resynchronization therapy
CRTP	cardiac resynchronization therapy pacing
CSA	central sleep apnoea
DCM	dilated cardiomyopathy
DT	deceleration time
ECG	electrocardiogram
EDV	estimated diastolic volume
EF	ejection fraction

EMPHASIZE-HF	Effect of Eplerenone in Chronic Systolic Heart Failure trial
EPHESUS	Eplerenone Post-acute myocardial infarction Heart Failure Efficacy and Survival Study
ESV	estimated systolic volume
GFR	glomerular filtration rate
HCM	hypertrophic cardiomyopathy
HFNEF	heart failure with a normal ejection fraction
IABP	intra-aortic balloon pump
ICD	implantable cardioverter defibrillator
JGA	juxtaglomerular apparatus
JVP	jugular venous pressure
LAVI	left atrial volume index
LV	left-ventricular
LVEDP	left-ventricular end-diastolic pressure
LVEDVI	left-ventricular end-diastolic volume index
LVEF	left-ventricular ejection fraction
LVIDs	left-ventricular internal diameter in systole
LVIDd	left-ventricular internal diameter in diastole
LVMI	left-ventricular mass index
LVNC	left-ventricular non-compaction
LVSD	left-ventricular systolic dysfunction
MD	macular densa
MERIT-HF	Metoprolol CR/XL Randomized Intervention Trial in Congestive Heart Failure
MMF	mycophenolate mofetil
mPCW	mean pulmonary capillary wedge pressure
NYHA	New York Heart Association
NHS	National Health Service (UK)
NICE	National Institute of Health and Clinical Excellence (UK)
NSAIDs	non-steroidal anti-inflammatory drugs
OSAHS	obstructive sleep apnoea/hypnoea syndrome
PEP-CHF	Perindopril in Elderly People with Chronic Heart Failure
%FS	percentage fractional shortening

PND	paroxysmal nocturnal dyspnoea
RAAS	renin-angiotensin-aldersterone system
RALES	Randomized Aldactone Evaluation Study
SDNN	standard deviation of normal to normal RR intervals over 24hrs
SHF	systolo-diastolic dysfunction
SNS	sympathetic nervous system
SOLVD	Studies of Left-Ventricular Dysfunction
TDI	tissue Doppler imaging
TTR	transthyretin
2D	two-dimensional
UK-HEART	United Kingdom Evaluation and Assessment of Risk Trial
VAD	ventricular assist device
Val-HeFT	Valsartan in Heart Failure Trial

Chapter 1

Aetiology and epidemiology of chronic heart failure

Iain Squire

> ### Key points
>
> - Principally due to the ageing population and improvements in outcome after myocardial infarction, chronic heart failure (CHF) is increasing in prevalence.
> - CHF is associated with a major detrimental effect on quality of life and life expectancy.
> - CHF may result from any number of cardiac pathologies; in western society, the main causes are ischaemic heart disease, hypertension and degenerative valve disease.
> - Less common aetiological conditions include toxins, infiltrative processes and familial cardiomyopathies.
> - In an individual patient, the "type" of CHF is best described in terms of the aetiology.

1.1 Aetiology of chronic heart failure

1.1.1 Background

It is often said that chronic heart failure (CHF) is a medical problem of epidemic proportions. While it may be difficult to make such a statement without danger of hyperbole, a number of facts about CHF are undeniably true. First, CHF is common, and is an important health-care issue in both general practice and hospital settings. Second, CHF is an important issue for patients suffering from the condition, being disabling and deadly: CHF is among the most common reasons for unplanned hospital admissions, and mortality from the condition is comparable to or worse than most of the common malignancies (see Chapter 4).

Third, CHF is costly, representing a large and growing drain on health-care resources. CHF has as great an impact upon quality of life as any other long-term condition and has an equally stark impact upon life expectancy. On this background, CHF has been the subject of intense scientific investigation over the last 20–30 years. As a result our understanding of the pathophysiology, aetiology, natural history, and prognosis of CHF has improved enormously.

It is important to recognise that CHF is not a disease entity in itself. Rather, CHF is a clinical syndrome, which is the consequence of a disease process, or combination of processes (discussed in Chapter 2). A clinically meaningful definition of CHF is that provided by the European Society of Cardiology (see Box 1.1). This emphasises the important issues, namely that appropriate symptoms should be present alongside objective evidence of left-ventricular dysfunction.

1.1.2 **CHF—aetiological conditions**

CHF may result from any number of pathological processes, which lead to abnormal cardiac structure, function or rhythm (see Box 1.2).

The principal factors contributing to prevalent heart failure vary with the population under study. In developing countries, rheumatic valvular heart disease, other infective causes such as trypanosomiasis, and nutritional deficiencies, are prevalent. In contrast, in industrialised societies, coronary heart disease and hypertension (with an increasingly important contribution from type 2 diabetes mellitus) are the main factors contributing to the development of CHF. Idiopathic aetiology, toxins (including alcohol), and atrial fibrillation are also important, with a variety of less common causes (e.g. amyloidosis, inherited cardiomyopathies, iron overload, peripartum cardiomyopathy) making lesser contributions (See Chapter 8 for detailed discussion of inherited cardiomyopathies).

Most conditions leading to the syndrome of CHF cause left-ventricular systolic dysfunction. Most such pathological processes will lead to left-ventricular dilatation in a large proportion of cases (discussed in Chapter 2). Specific conditions of the myocardium show a very different phenotype; in particular, infiltrative processes, such as amyloidosis, result in a restrictive cardiomyopathy with a small left ventricle.

In a proportion of patients with CHF, left-ventricular function appears to be preserved (discussed in detail in Chapter 9). This type of CHF is characteristically associated with hypertensive heart disease.

Box 1.1 ESC definition of heart failure

1. Symptoms of heart failure at rest or during exercise
2. Objective evidence of cardiac dysfunction at rest
3. Where the diagnosis remains in doubt, clinical response to treatment directed towards heart failure

Criteria 1 and 2 should be fulfilled in all cases

Box 1.2 Causes of heart failure

Myocardial Pathology
- Ischaemic heart disease
- Hypertrophic cardiomyopathy
  - Systemic hypertension
  - Inherited hypertrophic cardiomyopathy
- Restrictive cardiomyopathy
  - Infiltration
    — Amyloidosis
    — Sarcoidosis
    — Neoplasm
  - Storage disorders
    — Haemochromatosis
    — Fabry disease
    — Glycogen Storage diseases
  - Endomyocardial disease
    — Radiotherpy
    — Endomyocardial fibrosis
    — Carcinoid
- Dilated Cardiomyopathy
  - Inherited (familial) cardiomyopathy
  - Toxins
    — Alcohol
    — Chemotherapy
    — Iron or copper
    — Cocaine
  - Metabolic disorders
    — Endocrine disease (e.g. thyroid dysfunction)
    — Nutritional deficiency
    — Autoimmune disease
  - Peripartum cardiomyopathy
  - Neuromuscular disease
    — Friedreich's ataxia
    — Muscular dystrophy
  - Infectious
    — Parasitic (e.g. Chagas disease)
    — Viruses
    — HIV
    — Bacteria
- General
  - Valve disease
  - Pericardial disease (e.g. calcification, infiltration)
  - Arrhythmia
  - Peripartum cardiomyopathy

At its most extreme, this condition is associated with preserved contractile function in the presence of marked left-ventricular hypertrophy into the left-ventricular chamber. In an individual patient, the "type" of CHF is best described in terms of the aetiology.

Even among apparently similar populations, the contribution of a single condition or risk factor to the development of CHF varies considerably. This phenomenon can be explained by a number of factors (see Box 1.3).

As might be expected, the standard risk factors for the development of coronary artery disease are for the most part associated with increased risk of CHF. Thus, hypertension, tobacco smoking, diabetes mellitus, obesity, and family history of coronary disease are all relevant, in that identification and treatment of these may delay or prevent the development of hypertensive and coronary heart disease, and thus of CHF. Similarly, assessment of the aetiology of CHF will often help to define appropriate management for the individual patient. A recent helpful classification of CHF from stages A to D puts risk factors for coronary disease at the beginning of a continuum ending in advanced CHF (see Figure 1.1) once a patient enters a stage they cannot go back to an earlier point in the classification.

> ### Box 1.3 Difficulties in defining underlying aetiology in patients with CHF
>
> - The criteria upon which aetiology is defined may be incomplete. For instance, coronary artery disease may not have been overtly manifest, and will be missed unless objective investigation is undertaken. Similarly, aetiological hypertension may have "burned out" by the time CHF has developed.
> - Data based upon post-mortem information is highly selective, and fails to consider aetiology on a population basis.
> - The populations upon which observations are based vary from selected clinical trials participants to population-based cohorts.
> - The criteria upon which a risk factor is deemed present may change with time. This applies to consideration of hypertension, diabetes and dyslipidaemia as possible contributors to the development of CHF, the criteria by which each of these is defined having changed at least once over recent years.
> - Not infrequently, multiple risk factors coincide in any one patient, and it may be difficult to ascribe with confidence the main culprit. For instance, in a patient with CHF resulting from an acute myocardial infarction, with hypertension as the main identifiable risk factor, what is the contribution of coronary disease and high blood pressure to the development of CHF?

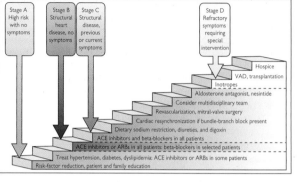

Figure 1.1 Staging of CHF, analogous to malignancy from high risk for CHF to advanced multisystem failure

Stage A
High risk with no symptoms

Stage B
Structural heart disease, no symptoms

Stage C
Structural disease, previous or current symptoms

Stage D
Refractory symptoms requiring special intervention

Hospice

VAD, transplantation

Inotropes

Aldosterone antagonist, nesintide

Consider multidisciplinary team

Revascularization, mitral-valve surgery

Cardiac resynchronization if bundle-branch block present

Dietary sodium restriction, diuretics, and digoxin

ACE inhibitors and beta-blockers in all patients

ACE inhibitors or ARBs in all patients: beta-blockers in selected patients

Treat hypertension, diabetes, dyslipidemia: ACE inhibitors or ARBs in some patients

Risk-factor reduction, patient and family education

1.1.3 **Inherited cardiomyopathies**

In assessing the aetiology of CHF in any single patient, the history is key. This will routinely consider standard risk factors such as prior myocardial infarction or history of hypertension and diabetes. In a young or middle-aged person in particular it is important to enquire about any family history of cardiomyopathy. This may not be initially apparent, and questions should be directed at establishing any family history of sudden cardiac, or unexplained death. A suspected or established inherited aetiology has implications for the patient's siblings and offspring. However, only a proportion of the gene mutations associated with these conditions can be detected with current technology.

1.1.4 **Chemotherapy and risk of CHF**

A further contribution to the changing demographics of CHF is exposure of a proportion of the population to "new" aetiological factors. In this context, increasing numbers of patients develop CHF as a consequence of exposure to chemotherapeutic agents for the treatment of malignancy. Anthracycline chemotherapy, administered as part of treatment for haematological malignancies or breast cancer, is of particular importance. The risk of cardiac damage in relation to anthracyclines is dose-related and hence, to some extent, predictable.

Some breast tumours are susceptible to chemotherapy with a humanised monoclonal antibody (trastuzumab (Herceptin)), against the HER2 protein. Trastuzumab has been identified as being associated with markedly increased risk of developing CHF, with approximately 10% of treated women developing some deterioration in left-ventricular

Figure 1.1 is reproduced with permission from Jessup M, Brozena S. 2003. Heart failure. *N. Engl. J. Med.*, **348**: 2007–18.

5

function, and 2–4% overt CHF. Trastuzumab also appears to sensitise the cardiomyocyte to the toxic effects of anthracyclines, and as such the two treatments should not be administered concurrently.

1.1.5 Is the aetiology of CHF changing?

The earliest epidemiological study of CHF was from the Framingham Heart Study, which reported the main aetiological factor to be hypertension in over 70% of cases. However the vast majority of epidemiological studies have failed to reproduce this finding. Indeed, more recent reports from Framingham indicate the proportion of prevalent CHF that is due to hypertension is falling, while that due to coronary disease is increasing. This trend may be in part due to earlier identification and better treatment of hypertension but also to better identification of causes of CHF other than hypertension, such as coronary heart disease.

1.2 Epidemiology of CHF

1.2.1 Background

Due in no little part to the increasing recognition of CHF as an important personal and public-health issue and to the associated volume of clinical research, the epidemiology of CHF in industrialised societies is well understood. Numerous studies from countries such as Australia, England, Scotland, Sweden, the Netherlands, and the USA have revealed a great deal about the burden of CHF in these societies. Importantly, these studies also tell us about trends in the epidemiology.

1.2.2 Incidence and prevalence of CHF

The incidence of CHF can be difficult to establish with certainty, relying upon the accurate identification of patients developing CHF for the first time. A number of population based epidemiological studies, and cohort-based prospective studies have addressed this issue. The overall incidence reported in these studies is between 1 and 5 cases per thousand population per annum. There are very few cases below the age of 45 years, increasing to 6–8 per thousand population per year at age 60–69. There is a steep rise in annual incidence to 15–20 per thousand for those aged 75 years or over and to over 25 per thousand in the very elderly (80+).

There is a male predominance in CHF up to the age of around 70 years, reflecting the higher incidence of coronary artery disease in men. Thereafter, the trend is reversed, and in terms of patients admitted to hospital with CHF, numbers are evenly split between men and women.

Over the last 30 years of the 20th century, hospital admission rates for CHF increased over threefold to over 30 per 1000 population per year. It appears that age-adjusted rates of hospital admission are decreasing, following several decades of steady increase. Whether this represents a reduction in new cases, or changes in the management of CHF, involving greater community-based care, is unclear. Data from the Framingham Heart Study suggest that between 1950 and 1990, the incidence of CHF declined slightly, particularly among women. However, in the context of an ageing population the number of hospital admissions with CHF continues to increase.

The prevalence of CHF is difficult to ascertain with accuracy, due to methodological differences among studies. Overall prevalence has been estimated at 1–2% of the adult population, this increases with age, affecting as many as 10% of individuals aged 65 years and over.

CHF accounts for a large proportion of activity in primary care, where the condition ranks second only to hypertension and alongside angina in terms of numbers of consultations. Current general-practitioner visits of approximately 90 per 1000 population per annum are projected to increase by over 30%, to 130, by the year 2020.

1.2.3 Economic cost of CHF

As might be expected from a highly prevalent condition, CHF is associated with significant health-care costs, estimated at approximately 2% of United Kingdom National Health Service spending in recent years. The major part of these costs relates to hospitalization. Importantly, proven pharmacological therapies make up only a very small proportion of the overall cost of CHF to the health-care budget in industrialised society.

On this background, CHF is currently regarded as a long-term condition for which attempts should be made to reduce hospitalizations, and thus reduce costs. The impact of such a strategy on prognosis for patients with CHF remains to be established. In the same context, the increasing application of device technology—namely implantable cardioverter defibrillator and cardiac resynchronization therapies (see Chapter 7)—may alter the balance of the overall cost of managing CHF.

1.2.4 Symptomatic or asymptomatic CHF

As the term "CHF" implies the presence of symptoms or physical signs, asymptomatic patients may be missed in some studies. Indeed, echocardiographic studies have suggested that approximately 50% of individuals with left-ventricular systolic dysfunction (LVSD) are asymptomatic.

A number of studies have assessed the feasibility of screening for asymptomatic LVSD. The cost-effectiveness of this approach is not fully established. However, targeting of high-risk groups (those with a history of coronary disease or an abnormal ECG) improves detection rate markedly. Detection of asymptomatic cases is worthwhile, as pharmacological therapy is effective in slowing progression to symptomatic

CHF. We recently conducted a study in which 1300 individuals with out a prior diagnosis of CHF underwent screening for the condition We assessed the utility of various natriuretic peptides, as well as clinical and historical features, in identifying patients with low left-ventricular ejection fraction. Table 1.1 indicates that gender, the presence of a major ECG abnormality (left-ventricular hypertrophy, Q-wave, left-bundle branch block, or atrial fibrillation), renal function, and a history of coronary heart disease were able to identify most such patients.

Table 1.1	Features showing low left-ventricular ejection fraction				
	Factor	Definite systolic heart failure (N = 17)		Definite and borderline systolic heart failure (N = 30)	
		Odds ratio	P value	Odds ratio	P value
BNP	Gender (male)	1.2	NS	4.2	0.012
	Creatinine	1.0	NS	1.0	NS
	major ECG abnormality	9.6	0.007	4.1	0.006
	BNP*	2.4	0.0005	2.7	0.0005
	Ischaemic heart history	3.9	0.027	2.5	0.075
N-BNP	Gender (male)	1.6	NS	3.8	0.009
	Creatinine	1.0	NS	1.0	NS
	major ECG abnormality	14.0	0.001	6.7	0.0005
	N-BNP*	1.5	0.002	1.4	0.0005
	Ischaemic heart history	4.3	0.008	2.9	0.016
N-ANP	Gender (male)	1.4	NS	2.9	0.037
	Creatinine	1.0	NS	1.0	NS
	major ECG abnormality	18.2	0.0005	9.5	0.0005
	N-ANP*	1.7	0.002	1.3	0.026
	Ischaemic heart history	5.9	0.001	4.0	0.001

* Odds ratio for 50% increase in peptide levels.

Table 1.1 is reproduced with permission from Ng LL, Loke IW, Davies JE, Geereanavar S, Khunti K, et al. 2005. Community screening for left-ventricular systolic dysfunction using plasma and urinary natriuretic peptides. J. Am. Coll. Cardiol., **45**: 1043–50.

1.2.5 **CHF with reduced, or normal, ejection fraction?**

The syndrome of CHF is largely associated with conditions leading to impaired left-ventricular function. Epidemiological and population based studies suggest that up to 50% of patients with CHF have this syndrome in the context of preserved left-ventricular ejection fractions (see Chapter 9 for detailed discussion of CHF with preserved ejection fraction).

The aetiology of CHF with preserved ejection fraction differs from that in those with reduced cardiac function. Preserved function CHF tends to be associated with a history of hypertension, rather than with coronary heart disease. Moreover, the vast majority of studies of pharmacological and non-pharmacological interventions in CHF have studied patients with impaired left-ventricular systolic function and reduced ejection fractions. To date, studies of such interventions in those with preserved systolic function have demonstrated at best marginal benefit. As a consequence, the evidence-base for the pharmacological treatment of CHF with preserved systolic function is limited.

Key references

McMurray, J.J.V., Pfeffer, M.A. (2005). Heart failure. *Lancet*, **365**, 1877–89.

Mosterd, A., Hoes, A.W. (2007). Clinical epidemiology of heart failure. *Heart*, **93**, 1137–46.

Fonarow, G.C., Heywood, J.T., Heidenreich, P.A., Lopatin, M., Yancy, C.W. (2007). Temporal trends in clinical characteristics, treatments, and outcomes for heart failure hospitalizations, 2002 to 2004: findings from Acute Decompensated Heart Failure National Registry (ADHERE). *Am. Heart J.*, **153**, 1021–7.

Jessup, M., Brozena, S. (2003). Heart failure. *N. Engl. J. Med.*, **348**, 2007–18.

Levy, D., Kenchaiah, S., Larson, M.G., *et al.* (2002). Long term trends in the incidence of and survival with heart failure. *N. Engl. J. Med.*, **347**, 1397–402.

Lloyd-Jones, D.L., Larson, M.G., Leip, E.P., *et al.* (2002). Lifetime risk for developing congestive heart failure: the Framingham heart study. *Circulation*, **102**, 3068–72.

Davis, R.C., Hobbs, F.D., Kenkre, J.E., *et al.* (2002). Prevalence of left-ventricular systolic dysfunction and heart failure in high risk patients: community based epidemiological study. *BMJ*, **325**, 1156–60.

Ng, L.L., Loke, I.W., Davies, J.E., *et al.* (2005). Community screening for left-ventricular systolic dysfunction using plasma and urinary natriuretic peptides. *J. Am. Coll. Cardiol.*, **45**, 1043–50.

Ng, L.L., Loke., I., Davies, J.E., *et al.* (2003). Identification of previously undiagnosed left-ventricular systolic dysfunction: community screening using natriuretic peptides and electrocardiography. *Eur. J. Heart Failure*, **5**, 775–82.

Chapter 2

Pathophysiology of systolic heart failure

Richard Cubbon and Ajay Shah

Key points

- Chronic heart failure (CHF) is a clinical syndrome in which pathological stress or injury is associated with a failure of cardiac performance to meet the metabolic demands of the body and therefore results in clinical symptoms.
- In the normal heart, cardiac output increases up to four fold during exercise; this response is diminished in CHF.
- Multiple intrinsic and extrinsic control mechanisms exist to optimise cardiac performance, both acutely and chronically, through modulation of cardiac physiology and structure.
- CHF is characterized by activation of a portfolio of compensatory mechanisms including activation of the renin-angiotensin-aldosterone and sympathetic nervous systems.
- An index cardiac insult may initiate maladaptive compensatory mechanisms instigating a vicious cycle of progressive myocardial damage, hence resulting in a deteriorating clinical syndrome of CHF.

Key terms

- Systole—the period of the cardiac cycle when ventricular activity occurs and blood is ejected
- Diastole—the period of the cardiac cycle when the heart fills with blood
- Cardiac cycle—the series of cardiac electromechanical events that comprise each beat
- Heart rate—the number of cardiac cycles per minute
- Chronotropy—modulation of heart rate
- Stroke volume—the volume of blood ejected from the heart during systole

- Inotropism—modulation of myocardial contractility
- Lusitropism—modulation of cardiac relaxation
- Cardiac output—the volume of blood pumped by the heart during 1 min
- Preload—the stretching force experienced by the myocardium prior to onset of contraction
- Afterload—the stretching force experienced by the myocardium during contraction
- Remodelling—cardiac structural and functional adaptation in response to chronic changes in workload

2.1 **Introduction**

The heart plays a central role in meeting the metabolic needs of all tissues by ensuring adequate circulation of blood through the vasculature. In the normal resting state this requires pumping the entire circulating volume of blood approximately once every minute. However, during times of increased metabolic demand, such as exercise, the heart must augment its pumping capacity significantly—up to four fold during heavy exercise. Chronic heart failure is a clinical syndrome in which pathological stress or injury is associated with a failure of cardiac performance to meet the metabolic demands of the body and therefore results in clinical symptoms. Mechanistically, the dominant problem is a loss of contractile reserve even though the signs and symptoms of the syndrome are often the result of "compensatory" pathways activated in response to this reduction in heart function.

In this chapter, we first outline the physiological pathways that facilitate acute and chronic alterations in cardiac function in response to increased demand, before discussing the response to pathological stress and the development of overt heart failure.

2.2 **Physiological regulation of cardiac contractile function**

Cardiac output, the volume of blood pumped per minute, is the product of heart rate and stroke volume (the volume of blood ejected from the left ventricle during each beat). An acute increase in cardiac output can be achieved through increases in heart rate or stroke volume or both, which are regulated by complex mechanisms intrinsic to the heart as well as extrinsic neurohormonal pathways. The heart can also undergo chronic changes in structure and function when faced with a persistent alteration in its workload. Before exploring

Table 2.1 Examples of heart failure aetiologies classified according to broad pathophysiological mechanisms

Myocardial disease	Elevated preload	Elevated afterload
Myocardial infarction	Mitral regurgitation	Aortic stenosis
Myocarditis	Aortic regurgitation	Systemic hypertension
Toxins (e.g. alcohol)	Intracardiac shunt	Aortic coarctation

the mechanisms that enable the heart to alter its work output, it is important to be familiar with the cardiac cycle—i.e. the repetitive pattern of cardiac electro-mechanical activity.

2.2.1 **The cardiac cycle**

With each beat of the heart a highly coordinated pattern of electrical activity spreads through the myocardium, which is ultimately responsible for the flow of blood from atrium to ventricle and then into the circulation (see Figure 2.1 and Figure 2.2). Originating in the sinoatrial node, the initial electrical discharge depolarises the atria resulting in their contraction (or systole). This electrical activity is then conducted to the ventricles via the atrioventricular node, through the ventricular myocardium by the His–Purkinje system. Ventricular systole commences with a period of rising pressure prior to ejection of blood—isovolumic contraction. Once the rising ventricular pressures exceed those of the aorta and pulmonary artery, respectively, blood is ejected into the systemic and pulmonary circulation.

A fall in left-ventricular pressure (or relaxation) leads to closure of the aortic valve when the pressure falls below aortic pressure, and this is followed by a period of isovolumic relaxation. Once ventricular pressure falls below atrial pressure, the ventricle starts to fill again with blood from the atrium. The phase of early rapid ventricular filling is significantly influenced by the rate of fall of actively developed pressure in the ventricular myocardium, which may induce a suction effect. The subsequent phase of ventricular filling is augmented by atrial systole. Both phases of filling are also influenced by the passive material properties of the ventricles, which determine their passive stiffness and therefore compliance. The term diastole generally refers to the filling phase of the cardiac cycle and does not strictly speaking include ventricular relaxation. However, ventricular relaxation has the potential to influence diastolic filling, as discussed above.

Appropriate pump function of the heart is dependent upon both systolic and diastolic function since ejection of blood is inextricably linked to filling of the heart. Indeed, as outlined in Chapter 9, many patients with heart failure have relatively preserved systolic function suggesting that the primary defect may lie in diastolic function.

Figure 2.1 Schema of the cardiac conduction system

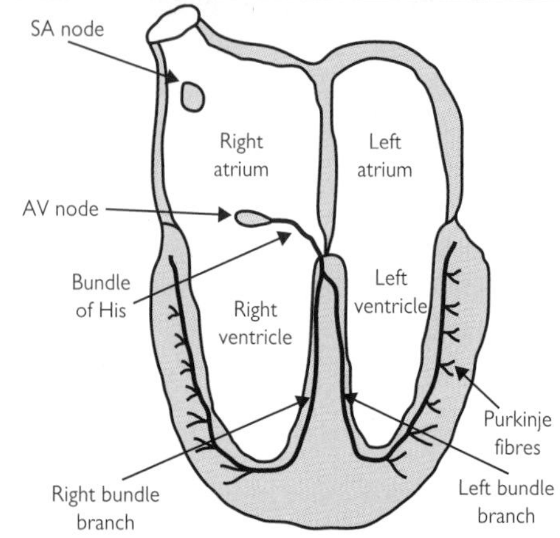

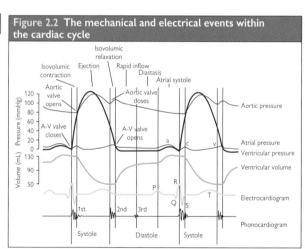

Figure 2.2 The mechanical and electrical events within the cardiac cycle

2.2.2 Acute intrinsic regulation of heart function

Four main inter-related factors influence the contractile function of the heart in the short term under physiological conditions, namely (a) it's intrinsic contractility or inotropic state, (b) the preload (or volume load) on the heart, which is determined largely by venous return and

Figure 2.1 is reproduced with permission from Wikipedia.

which influences end-diastolic volume, (c) the afterload (or pressure load or resistance) against which the heart ejects blood, and (d) the heart rate.

The inotropic state of the heart is affected by 1) factors intrinsic to the cardiomyocyte (such as muscle energetics, excitation-contraction coupling and myofilament properties), 2) the coronary blood supply, and 3) by extrinsic pathways. Changes in preload of the heart directly link stroke volume to venous return through the Frank–Starling relationship. The seminal studies of Otto Frank and Ernest Starling showed that increases in venous return to the heart resulted in cardiac chamber stretching followed by enhanced myocardial contractility and therefore stroke volume. While debate still persists regarding the precise mechanisms of this effect, a major mechanism at a molecular level is a length-dependent enhancement of the contractile response of muscle myofilaments to systolic calcium (so-called myofilament calcium responsiveness). In other words, the strength of contraction of heart muscle or of the ventricular chamber is proportional to the initial muscle length or chamber volume (end-diastolic volume) respectively. This relationship persists up to a plateau beyond which further increments in venous return result in a decline in stroke volume, probably due to overstretching of the cardiac contractile apparatus (see Figure 2.3). It is important to note that the relationship between preload and stroke volume is itself affected by other regulatory mechanisms. For example, an increase in inotropic state results in a steeper rise in stroke volume per unit increase in preload.

The effect of afterload on heart function can best be understood by considering that there is an inverse relationship between the heart muscle's ability to develop force (and therefore elevate ventricular pressure) and its ability to shorten (and therefore eject blood—i.e. stroke volume). The level of intraventricular pressure that is developed is directly linked to the afterload so that elevation of afterload is accompanied by a decrease in stroke volume whereas a reduction in afterload leads to increased stroke volume. An increase in heart rate increases the inotropic state of the healthy heart through the positive force-frequency relationship, the cellular basis of which mainly involves an enhanced cycling of calcium within cardiomyocytes at higher heart rate.

Beyond optimising cardiac output, the intrinsic mechanisms that alter heart function also impact on its workload and therefore energy utilisation. The workload of ventricular muscle is related to its wall stress or the force developed per unit muscle tissue. The factors influencing wall stress are given by Laplace's law which states that wall stress is directly proportional to the pressure within the ventricular cavity and its diameter (or volume) and is inversely proportional to chamber wall thickness. Therefore, increases in both preload and afterload increase wall stress by increasing ventricular volume and pressure, respectively, whereas an increase in wall thickness decreases wall stress. The responses of the heart to chronic increases in wall stress are central to understanding the development of myocardial dysfunction in the setting of systolic heart failure (*see later*).

2.2.3 **Extrinsic control mechanisms**

Enhanced sympathetic nervous system (SNS) activity is perhaps the most potent extrinsic means of augmenting cardiac output via both its positive chronotropic and positive inotropic effects. Parasympathetic influences on the heart are largely mediated by modulation of sympathetic tone although the possibility of direct parasympathetic effects is also debated. A wide range of neurohormonal mechanisms can also influence heart function both through effects on circulating volume and vascular tone (i.e. extracardiac effects) and direct effects on the heart. An increase in circulating blood volume increases venous return and therefore preload while an increase in systemic vasoconstriction increases afterload. The factors regulating circulating volume and peripheral vascular tone include the renin-angiotensin-aldosterone system (RAAS), the autonomic nervous system, circulating hormones and peptides (such as natriuretic peptides, glucocorticoids, and arginine vasopressin), and locally generated autocrine/paracrine factors (such as nitric oxide, prostanoids, and endothelins)—which act at many different levels within the body, including the brain, kidneys, and vasculature. In addition to the systemic effects of these neurohumoral and autocrine/paracrine factors, research over the last two decades has increasingly established that many of these agents may be locally generated within the heart itself and exert direct effects on contractile function.

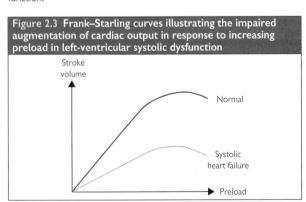

Figure 2.3 Frank–Starling curves illustrating the impaired augmentation of cardiac output in response to increasing preload in left-ventricular systolic dysfunction

2.3 **Chronic physiological adaptation**

Besides the mechanisms that allow rapid modulation of heart function in response to varying workload, there is also the physiological capacity to alter structure and function (called remodelling) in the face of a chronic alteration in heart workload (or wall stress). Perhaps the best physiological examples of heart remodelling are the changes in structure and function that occur in healthy athletes. Adaptation to chronic isotonic exercise (e.g. long-distance running) usually involves an increase in end-diastolic volume, which may serve to facilitate large increases in stroke volume during exercise through enhanced utilisation of the Frank–Starling response (or preload reserve). In addition, there is also some thickening of the ventricular wall (hypertrophy), which can be considered adaptive because it serves to reduce the wall stress that is increased with increasing volume (by Laplace's law). Adaptation to chronic isometric exercise (e.g. weight lifting) usually involves mainly an increase in wall thickness since in this case the increased work is largely due to increased pressure (afterload) rather than volume (preload).

Whereas ventricular hypertrophy or dilatation or both also occur in myocardial diseases leading to heart failure, key attributes of physiological remodelling are a concomitant increase in myocardial vascularisation and the absence of fibrosis. Indeed, elucidation of the molecular and cellular basis for the differences between physiological and pathological heart remodelling is a major research goal, the answer to which may open up novel therapeutic possibilities.

2.4 **Cardiac responses to pathological stress or injury**

Although a diverse spectrum of myocardial pathology can cause heart dysfunction, the responses to such insults are quite restricted in their variety such that the clinical phenotype of the heart failure syndrome is relatively uniform regardless of the underlying primary cause. The commonest causes of systolic heart failure are either myocardial infarction (where loss of myocardium results in a chronic increase in workload in the non-infarcted myocardium) or conditions that induce chronic increases in pressure or volume load on the heart (see Table 2.1).

2.4.1 **Acute responses**

When heart function is reduced by injury or stress (e.g. acute myocardial infarction), the same acute mechanisms that are normally utilised to augment cardiac output in the physiological setting are initially recruited. An increase in SNS activation and in heart rate serves to augment cardiac output via positive inotropy and a steepening of the Frank–Starling relationship (see Figure 2.3). Systemic neurohumoral pathways are also activated to increase circulating volume, which serves to augment venous return and therefore maintain cardiac output through recruitment of preload reserve (the Frank–Starling response). Systemic vasoconstriction allows the maintenance of blood pressure (although at the cost of increased afterload on the heart). Collectively, these adaptive responses will often normalise cardiac output at rest and thus avoid the development of symptoms, at least in the short-term. However, an important consequence of the use of these mechanisms to maintain resting cardiac output is that the overall reserve available for further increases in cardiac output is reduced. Therefore, the exercise capacity of such patients may be significantly reduced which at least in part explains the exertional nature of many symptoms of heart failure.

2.4.2 **Chronic remodelling**

Whilst the early compensatory response to abnormal cardiac contractility or load primarily involves functional responses in biochemical pathways, observational studies have shown that cardiac structure can also progressively change. These structural modifications are intricately linked with the ongoing physiological adaptations in many neurohormonal systems that develop in response to a persistent contractile deficit. Augmented systemic and local activity of many cytokine or growth-factor families (e.g. the SNS and RAAS) stimulates diverse cellular and extracellular structural modification. In broad terms, such cardiomyocyte hypertrophy and modified extracellular matrix turnover impact upon myocardial wall and chamber dimensions; these changes may initially assist the maintenance of adequate stroke volume and myocardial load.

The nature of compensatory structural modification, or remodelling, is dependent on the specific cardiac insult, though it is broadly predictable according to Laplace's law (see Figure 2.4). For example, aortic stenosis elevates left-ventricular afterload and so this chamber must generate more force to maintain stroke volume; to normalise the elevated wall stress generalised left-ventricular hypertrophy develops. The pattern of hypertrophy in this case is not associated with myocyte stretching and is termed concentric. In contrast, mitral regurgitation elevates left-ventricular preload and the so the chamber dilates as expected from the Frank–Starling relationship. Wall stress is elevated by chamber dilatation and so generalised hypertrophy again ensues; this pattern of hypertrophy with chamber dilatation is referred to as *eccentric*. Equally, myocardial infarction often alters cardiac load, though this involves regional disturbances in preload and afterload, resulting in more complex structural adaptation.

Progressive myocardial injury with an insidious decline in contractile function can result in incremental activation of these processes, and so functional compensation. When myocardial injury is severe, compensatory mechanisms may fail to adequately augment cardiac output, in which case heart failure ensues. In this scenario regulatory mechanisms may continue to elevate preload beyond the plateau phase of the Frank–Starling relationship and so cardiac output falls below its potential maximum. This elevation in venous return, and therefore venous pressure, can also worsen matters by precipitating pulmonary and peripheral oedema. The severity of these adverse outcomes depends upon the degree of myocardial injury and the adequacy of compensatory response. Furthermore, the chronology of myocardial injury is important in determining response. As outlined next, a slowly progressive insult is generally better tolerated than an acute insult of similar magnitude; this is because compensatory mechanisms can progressively adapt cardiac function to maintain sufficient cardiac output.

2.5 **Progression to cardiac failure**

Clearly some myocardial insults can be adapted for by functional and structural compensatory responses, resulting in an asymptomatic period; such adjustments are undoubtedly beneficial over the short term in that they maintain life. When abnormal cardiac function persists, long-term activation of these adaptations occurs, yet many patients who initially compensate will later develop progressive heart failure, despite suffering no further overt cardiac injury. This observation led to speculation that compensatory responses may become maladaptive over the longer term and so heralded a new era in our conceptualisation of heart failure pathophysiology. In this paradigm, persistent activation of biochemical and structural compensatory responses further impairs cardiac contractility, hence initiating a self-perpetuating cycle of progressive cardiac injury (see Figure 2.5).

2.5.1 **Neurohormonal mechanisms**

Persistent neurohormonal stimulation has wide-ranging effects upon the cardiomyocyte, its supporting matrix and the many other cell types within the myocardium. Chronic catecholamine release stimulates myocyte hypertrophy and interstitial fibrosis; moreover, the SNS is also a potent stimulus for myocyte death through apoptosis and necrosis. Furthermore, it induces the transcription of fetal genes, which aids energy conservation, but at the expense of reduced cellular contractile potential. Chronic catecholamine stimulation also results in adrenoreceptor downregulation and hyperphosphorylation of many proteins in its intracellular signalling pathways, so reducing their capacity to transduce signals. This severely limits the capacity of adrenergic compensatory mechanisms to augment cardiac output in future periods of acute haemodynamic stress. Calcium metabolism, crucial to excitation–contraction coupling within the myocyte, is also

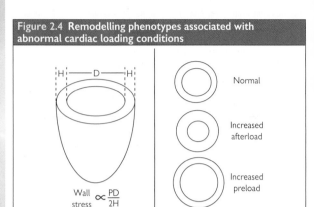

Figure 2.4 **Remodelling phenotypes associated with abnormal cardiac loading conditions**

Wall stress $\propto \dfrac{PD}{2H}$

Normal

Increased afterload

Increased preload

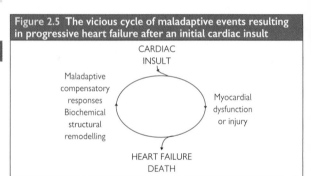

Figure 2.5 **The vicious cycle of maladaptive events resulting in progressive heart failure after an initial cardiac insult**

CARDIAC INSULT

Maladaptive compensatory responses
Biochemical structural remodelling

Myocardial dysfunction or injury

HEART FAILURE DEATH

disordered in response to a number of neurohormonal cascades, resulting in impaired contractility and enhanced arrhythmia risk.

The SNS is also closely linked with the RAAS given its capacity to stimulate renal renin release (see Chapter 5); importantly the RAAS is equally capable of persistent activation independent of the SNS. Historically, RAAS activation was only thought to occur in response to renal hypoperfusion, with systemic release of its mediators. However, local myocardial production of angiotensin and aldosterone, in response to elevated wall stress, now appears to be more important in the pathophysiology of heart failure. As outlined beforehand, the system stimulates vasoconstriction and renal sodium retention, so maintaining blood pressure and augmenting preload. However, angiotensin and aldosterone, in particular, have direct effects upon cardiac cells, which mediate the negative impact of chronic RAAS stimulation after cardiac injury. RAAS activity promotes myocardial fibrosis (collagen deposition), cardiomyocyte hypertrophy, and cellular apoptosis or necrosis, which results in a stiffened, hypocontractile myocardium. It also appears that the strength of the extracellular collagen matrix deteriorates as a result of increased degradatory enzyme release, which in conjunction with cardiomyocyte death may contribute to progressive ventricular dilatation.

Other less well explored neurohormonal systems that may contribute to the progression of heart failure include arginine vasopressin (or antidiuretic hormone; ADH) and endothelin. The former is a potent stimulus for renal water retention and so raises preload; the latter is in some ways similar to angiotensin II in that it potently vasoconstricts and promotes cardiomyocyte death along with myocardial fibrosis. Natriuretic peptides, including atrial and brain natriuretic peptides, are somewhat unusual in the spectrum of neurohormonal responses in that they appear to protect from the negative effects of other upregulated systems. Released from the myocardium in response to stretch, they promote renal sodium excretion, vasodilate, and interfere with aldosterone synthesis.

2.5.2 Structural remodelling

Beyond neurohormones, a diverse array of inflammatory cytokines is also upregulated during the development of heart failure; these have diverse effects including stimulation of cardiomyocyte hypertrophy, apoptosis or necrosis, along with impairing EC coupling. The myocardium can produce such compounds although many other sources exist and the reason for their upregulation in heart failure requires further investigation. Many of these cytokines, in combination with the RAAS and endothelin, also impair normal function of the vascular endothelium potentially resulting in reduced myocardial perfusion and so worsening contractile dysfunction; systemic vasoconstriction also increases cardiac afterload. Oxidative stress, a term describing excess production of reactive oxygen species or deficiency of antioxidants, has also been implicated in the progression of heart failure. Reactive oxygen species are able to damage proteins and nucleic acids; as such they can impair myocyte energy generation, interfere with excitation–contraction coupling, precipitate myocyte apoptosis, promote fibrosis, and impair endothelial function. Multiple sources of reactive oxygen species become active during the progression to clinical heart failure.

Collectively, chronic activation of the biochemical systems discussed above results in further important alterations at a whole organ level. Whilst some aspects of myocardial structural remodelling may appear useful, the net impact is detrimental to the efficiency of cardiac work. As the ventricle dilates it tends to lose its elliptical form, instead adopting a spherical morphology. The combination of ventricular

21

dilatation and abnormal geometry displaces the atrioventricular valvular apparatus resulting in functional incompetence (mitral or tricuspid regurgitation); this elevates ventricular preload, initiating a further detrimental cycle of cardiac injury. Furthermore, elevated cardiac load reduces efficiency and so increases myocardial oxygen demand—in combination with increased wall stress this may promote subendo-cardial ischaemia, again reducing cardiac contractility. Relatively recently it has also been noted that remodelling is often associated with left-ventricular contractile dysynchrony—individual myocardial segments contract at subtly different times, which again reduces contractile efficiency.

2.6 **Conclusion**

It is clear that numerous biochemical and structural changes occur in the transition from an initial cardiac insult to clinically manifest cardiac failure. The paradigm outlined beforehand involving an index cardiac insult followed by a vicious cycle of maladaptive compensatory responses and structural/functional remodelling is attractive. However, as outlined in later chapters, contemporary therapeutic strategies which interfere with many of the proposed causative biochemical pathways fail to completely retard disease progression in the majority of patients. Our understanding of heart failure has advanced dramati-cally since the work of Frank and Starling, though many uncertainties remain and novel concepts of disease progression will be required.

Key references

Berk, B.C., Fujiwara, K., Lehoux, S. (2007). ECM remodelling in hypertensive heart disease. *J. Clin. Invest.*, **117**, 568–75.

Chen, H.H., Schrier, R.W. (2006). Pathophysiology of volume overload in acute heart failure syndromes. *Am. J. Med.*, **119**, S11–6.

Mann, D.L. (2004). Basic mechanisms of left-ventricular remodelling: the contribution of wall stress. *J. Card. Fail.*, **10**, S202–6.

Mann, D.L., Bristow, M.R. (2005). Mechanisms and models in heart failure: the biomechanical model and beyond. *Circulation*, **111**, 2837–49.

Opie, L.H., Commerford, P.J., Gerch, B.J., Pfeffer, M.A. (2006). Controversies in ventricular remodelling. *Lancet*, **367**, 356–67.

Schrier, R.W., Abraham, W.T. (1999). Hormones and hemodynamics in heart failure. *N. Engl. J. Med.*, **341**, 577–85.

Seddon, M., Looi, Y.H., Shah, A.M. (2007). Oxidative stress and redox signalling in cardiac hypertrophy and heart failure. *Heart*, **93**, 903–7.

Chapter 3

Investigation of patients with suspected chronic heart failure

Ninian N. Lang and David E. Newby

Key Points

- Heart failure may be suspected on the basis of symptoms and signs but requires the use of objective tests to confirm the diagnosis.
- As well as confirming the diagnosis, the assessment of patients with suspected heart failure should also define its severity, aetiology, and any precipitants of decompensation.
- The electrocardiogram has powerful negative predictive value in patients with suspected heart failure, whilst the measurement of atrial or brain natriuretic peptides is gaining favour as a 'rule-out' blood test.
- The echocardiogram remains the most important first-line test in patients with suspected heart failure although other imaging modalities are often indicated, including cardiac magnetic resonance imaging and cardiac catheterisation.

3.1 Background

Whilst asymptomatic left-ventricular dysfunction can be an incidental finding, symptoms reported by patients may raise the possibility of chronic heart failure (CHF), especially in the presence of typical physical signs. However, none of the symptoms or signs of CHF are specific for this syndrome and clinical suspicion must be confirmed with the use of objective tests. The assessment of patients with suspected heart failure should be comprehensive and not only establish its presence but also define its severity, attempt to elicit its underlying aetiology and identify relevant precipitants. By making this thorough evaluation it should be possible to formulate an appropriately tailored therapeutic strategy and make an approximate prognostic assessment (see Chapter 4).

3.2 Symptoms

Patients may be asymptomatic at rest and, indeed, resting indices of cardiac function are usually within the normal range unless the patient is put under physiological stress. The main symptoms of CHF are dyspnoea, fatigue, and peripheral oedema.

3.2.1 Dyspnoea

Dyspnoea is the most common presenting complaint in patients with CHF. It can manifest simply as breathlessness upon exertion but as severity increases patients may describe orthopnoea, paroxysmal nocturnal dyspnoea (PND), and shortness of breath at rest.

In those who are only breathless upon exertion, an attempt to quantify the exertion required to precipitate breathlessness should be made and enquiry regarding exercise tolerance. For those with severe symptoms, simple tasks such as washing or dressing may provoke dyspnoea and interference with activities of daily living should be assessed.

Whilst symptoms of dyspnoea do not correlate well with measures of left-ventricular performance, these symptoms are useful as an indicator of disease status or response to therapy in individual patients. Effort tolerance may be graded using the New York Heart Association (NYHA) classification (see Table 3.1) which has been used in most clinical trials in CHF and is a useful independent predictor of survival.

3.2.2 Fatigue

Patients with heart failure may complain of fatigue and weakness. Fatigue can be difficult to quantify, and often patients find it difficult to separate symptoms of fatigue from those of dyspnoea. The cause of fatigue is usually multifactorial but is often secondary to low cardiac output and poor tissue perfusion. Other factors include altered metabolism within skeletal muscle, elevated circulating cytokine concentrations, excessive activation of the neuroendocrine system, and deconditioning of skeletal muscles.

Table 3.1 New York Heart Association (NYHA) classification of heart failure

I	No limitation of physical activity
II	Slight limitation of physical activity—symptoms with ordinary levels of exertion (e.g. walking upstairs)
III	Marked limitation of physical activity—symptoms with minimal levels of exertion (e.g. dressing)
IV	Symptoms at rest

3.2.3 Oedema

Ankle swelling is often one of the first manifestations of CHF. However, some patients never develop peripheral oedema despite severe cardiac failure. Patients with symptoms of right-sided heart failure may complain of abdominal swelling secondary to ascites or pain in the right upper quadrant of the abdomen caused by hepatomegaly and stretch of the liver capsule. Oedema of the gastrointestinal tract may induce symptoms of nausea, anorexia, and bloating.

3.2.4 Cerebral symptoms

Symptoms such as confusion, disorientation, and mood changes may be reported in advanced heart failure and are particularly associated with hyponatraemia. These may be the presenting symptoms of heart failure in the elderly. Sleep disturbance may be associated with ventilatory abnormalities including Cheyne–Stokes respiration and sleep apnoea, which may be reported by the patient's partner.

3.2.5 Identification of aetiology and precipitants

As discussed in Chapter 1, cardiac ischaemia remains the most common cause of heart failure in the developed world. However, the history should encompass the possibility of alternative aetiologies and should identify potential precipitants of decompensation (see Table 3.2).

Table 3.2 Aetiologies and potential causes of decompensation of heart failure	
Aetiology of heart failure	Precipitants of decompensation
Ischaemic heart disease	Inappropriate reduction of medication
Hypertension	Myocardial ischaemia or infarction
Valvular heart disease	Cardiac arrhythmia
Infective	Systemic infection or unrelated illness
• viral	Pulmonary thromboembolism
• septic	High-output states
Alcohol	• anaemia
Idiopathic dilated cardiomyopathy	• pregnancy
Familial cardiomyopathies	• thyrotoxicosis
Infiltration	• Paget's disease
• amyloid	• systemic arterio-venous fistulae
• sarcoid	Cardiotoxins
• haemochromatosis	• alcohol
Collagen vascular disease	• cocaine

Table 3.2 (Contd.)	
Peripartum	Inappropriate medication
Chemotherapy	• NSAIDS (salt or water retention)
Radiotherapy	• negatively inotropic drugs
Metabolic/endocrine/nutritional	
• phaeochromocytoma	
• hypothyroidism	
• severe thiamine deficiency (beri-beri)	
Congenital heart disease	
Persistent tachycardia	

3.3 Signs

The general appearance of the patient with suspected heart failure can provide useful clues to the severity and duration of cardiac dysfunction. Generalised wasting with skeletal muscle loss (cardiac cachexia) indicates severe, late-stage heart failure but the majority of patients are of normal appearance and not breathless at rest.

3.3.1 Cardiovascular

In severe heart failure the pulse may be of low volume and the peripheries cool and cyanosed as a result of peripheral vasoconstriction. Pulsus alternans is indicative of a failing left ventricle and manifests as a regular rhythm with an alternating strong and weak pulse. Alternatively, the patient may be in atrial fibrillation or tachycardic, especially during periods of decompensation. Blood pressure is usually low as a result of poor cardiac output and the effects of cardiac medication but may be normal or high, especially if hypertension is the underlying cause of heart failure.

Raised jugular venous pressure (JVP) is an important finding and appropriate assessment is very helpful for the guidance of diuretic dosage. However, tricuspid regurgitation caused by right-ventricular dilatation is frequently found in patients with heart failure and is associated with giant 'V waves' that obscure the utility of JVP as an index of right atrial pressure. In patients with mild right heart failure, the JVP may be normal at rest but rise with the application of firm pressure to the right upper quadrant of the abdomen (hepatojugular reflux).

Left-ventricular dilatation causes a diffuse, laterally displaced apex beat and a right-ventricular heave may be appreciated if pulmonary artery pressures are elevated or right heart failure has occurred. Cardiac auscultation may reveal a third heart sound or 'gallop rhythm' which is usually only audible in the presence of severe left-ventricular dysfunction and dilatation. It is associated with a poor prognosis but may disappear with treatment. Cardiac auscultation may also reveal the pansystolic murmur of mitral regurgitation which may be caused by organic valve disease or, more commonly, by secondary dilatation of the mitral valve annulus. The presence of any murmur may indicate valvular pathology, or a septal defect, in the aetiology of the patient's heart failure.

3.3.2 Respiratory

Patients with decompensated or severe heart failure may be tachypnoeic at rest. Fine bibasal crepitations may be heard and are the result of transudation of fluid from the vasculature into alveoli and the airways. However, crepitations are an unreliable sign of pulmonary oedema. If present, pleural effusions are usually bilateral but a unilateral effusion caused by heart failure tends to be found on the right side.

3.3.3 Oedema

Oedema is a cardinal feature of cardiac failure but has many other causes and does not correlate well with systemic venous pressure. It is commonly found at the ankles in mobile patients but often accumulates at the sacrum in bed-bound patients. It should be noted that peripheral oedema only develops after at least four litres of fluid have been gained. Patients with prominent signs of right heart failure may have ascites in addition to peripheral oedema.

3.3.4 Abdominal

Right heart failure causes hepatic congestion and smooth, tender hepatomegaly may be palpable and is sometimes associated with jaundice. Pulsatile hepatomegaly is found in association with tricuspid regurgitation.

3.4 Investigations

The investigation of patients with suspected heart failure should not only confirm the diagnosis but should also make an objective assessment of its severity and aetiology. Together with the identification of relevant comorbidity, complications, and precipitants, this information is vital to the selection of an appropriate therapeutic strategy and to monitor the response to it.

3.4.1 Clinical haematology and biochemistry

Anaemia can exacerbate cardiac failure and, occasionally, is the cause of it. It increases the metabolic demand of the heart and is a common finding in patients with advanced heart failure, in whom it is associated with an adverse prognosis. Macrocytosis may suggest alcohol or vitamin deficiency as either an aetiological or exacerbating factor.

Assessment of renal function is of particular importance as renal failure may masquerade as cardiac failure. In addition, severe heart failure itself is often associated with renal hypoperfusion and consequent renal dysfunction. Serum electrolyte balance is also frequently disturbed either as a consequence of the disease or, more commonly, as a result of treatment with diuretics and antagonists of the renin–angiotensin–aldosterone axis. Both hyponatraemia and hypokalaemia are adverse prognostic indicators in patients with heart failure.

Plasma fasting-glucose and lipid profile should be checked to detect the presence of diabetes mellitus and dyslipidaemias—both significant risk factors for coronary artery disease and heart failure. Both hypothyroidism and hyperthyroidism may go unrecognised and thyroid function tests should be checked in all patients.

Liver function tests may be abnormal as a result of hepatic congestion caused by cardiac failure. Alternatively, deranged liver function may suggest other potential aetiologies including alcohol excess or haemochromatosis and, therefore, iron binding capacity should be defined. Viral serology should be checked when the aetiology of heart failure is unclear and urinary metanephrines can help in the diagnosis of an underlying phaeochromcytoma. Heart failure as a result of cardiac sarcoidosis may be suggested by elevated serum angiotensin-converting enzyme and calcium concentrations. Cardiac enzymes should be measured at times of decompensation if myocardial ischaemia or infarction is a likely precipitant.

There has been a great deal of interest in the search for plasma biomarkers of heart failure and both atrial and brain natriuretic peptides appear to be relatively sensitive for its identification. They may be elevated in other conditions, including left-ventricular hypertrophy, and their specificity is limited. Therefore, their measurement has been proposed as a 'rule-out' test with the presence of a 'low-normal' concentration of natriuretic peptide (in an untreated patient) essentially excluding a diagnosis of heart failure. However, it is unclear whether measurement of the natriuretic peptides can improve upon the negative predictive value of a normal electrocardiogram and, on the whole, their measurement is confined to research use.

3.4.2 **Electrocardiogram**

Patients with heart failure rarely have a normal electrocardiogram and a normal electrocardiogram (ECG) carries a negative predictive value of approximately 98%.

The ECG can provide important clues to the underlying aetiology of the cardiac failure. For example, pathological Q waves and ST segment or T-wave changes suggest the presence of ischaemic heart disease. There may be ECG signs of left-ventricular hypertrophy in patients with hypertension, aortic stenosis and hypertrophic cardiomyopathy. Low voltage QRS complexes may be seen in hypothyroidism, amyloidosis and in the presence of a pericardial effusion. Pericardial effusion may also be associated with electrical alternans where the amplitude of the QRS complex changes with alternate beats due to the oscillation of the heart within the pericardial fluid.

The ECG may also provide evidence of conduction problems or arrhythmia. Bradycardia or complete heart block can exacerbate heart failure and may be a result of organic conduction system disease or drug side effects. Atrial arrhythmias are particularly common and may either be a cause or a consequence of heart failure. Some ECG findings, including atrial fibrillation, are associated with a worse prognosis. Similarly, left bundle branch block is associated with a worse outcome and these patients should be further assessed for their potential to benefit from cardiac resynchronization therapy (see Chapter 7 for details).

Ambulatory ECG monitoring is useful for the assessment of patients with symptoms suggestive of paroxysmal arrhythmia. In patients with atrial fibrillation, it provides a measure of rate control over a prolonged period.

3.4.3 **Chest X-ray**

The chest X-ray is a poor discriminator in chronic heart failure. Indeed, a normal cardiothoracic ratio has low sensitivity and specificity for the detection of heart failure and is normal in around 40–50% of patients with left-ventricular dysfunction. The relationship between haemodynamic and pulmonary vascular abnormalities are variable and some patients with severe heart failure may not have X-ray features of pulmonary venous congestion or oedema despite very high pulmonary capillary pressures. However, the chest X-ray can be useful for monitoring response to therapy, disease progression and the presence of ongoing pulmonary oedema (see Figure 3.1). It may also identify non-cardiac causes of breathlessness.

Classic chest X-ray features of cardiac failure:
- cardiomegaly (cardiothoracic ratio >0.5)
- upper lobe venous diversion
- 'Kerley B lines'
- fluid in horizontal fissure
- bilateral alveolar oedema inc. 'bats wing' perihilar shadowing
- pleural effusion (bilateral or R > L)
- peribronchial cuffing

Chest X-ray features providing clues to the aetiology:
- prominent hilar vessels (pulmonary hypertension)
- bulging left heart border with retrosternal 'double density' (left-ventricular aneurysm)

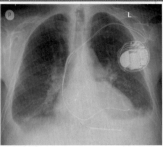

Note the presence of cardiomegaly, bilateral pleural effusions, bilateral alveolar oedema with perihilar shadowing, upper-lobe venous diversion, fluid in the horizontal fissure, and peribronchial cuffing.

- left atrial enlargement (mitral valve disease)
- pericardial calcification (constrictive pericarditis)
- valvular calcification (valvular heart disease)
- rib notching (coarctation of the aorta)

3.4.4 Echocardiography

The echocardiogram is the most important investigation for heart failure as it can detect the presence, the aetiology, and the severity of heart failure. Echocardiography can provide measures of left-ventricular function that include left-ventricular end diastolic diameter, shortening fraction, and ejection fraction (see Figure 3.2). Left-ventricular systolic function is considered to be impaired when the ejection fraction is less than 0.50.

Whilst global impairment of systolic function can be seen as a result of severe ischaemic heart disease, this pattern of dysfunction is particularly associated with a global insult to the heart and is characteristic of dilated cardiomyopathy. The presence of distinct areas of impaired myocardial contractility with large areas of normal contraction is suggestive of underlying coronary artery disease.

Echocardiography also provides useful information regarding diastolic function, wall thickness, and pulmonary-artery pressure. Various structural conditions associated with heart failure, such as valvular disease, left-ventricular hypertrophy, and pericardial disease including pericardial effusion, may be readily identified.

Stress echocardiography (dobutamine or exercise) can be useful for the detection of ischaemia as a cause of heart failure. It is a useful tool for the assessment of myocardial viability in the presence of marked hypokinesia or akinesia, especially if revascularisation is under consideration.

Figure 3.2 Echocardiogram of a patient with heart failure

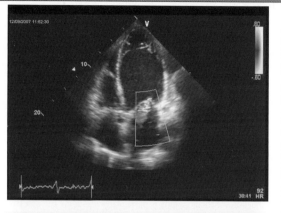

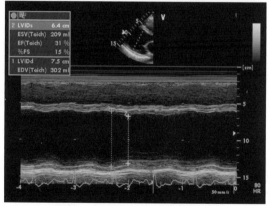

2-dimensional (2D) apical four chamber view demonstrating a grossly dilated left-ventricle and functional mitral regurgitation; B) M-mode imaging through the left-ventricular cavity demonstrating severe impairment of left-ventricular systolic function. LVIDs = left-ventricular internal diameter in systole; ESV = estimated systolic volume; EF = ejection fraction; %FS = percentage fractional shortening; LVIDd = left-ventricular internal diameter in diastole; EDV = estimated diastolic volume.

3.4.5 Exercise testing

Bicycle or treadmill exercise testing can provide an objective marker of exercise capacity and is especially useful when coronary artery disease is a likely cause of cardiac failure. There is, however, poor correlation between achieved exercise duration and left-ventricular ejection fraction. Simultaneous measurement of peak oxygen uptake may be used to make an assessment of prognosis and for the selection of patients who may benefit from cardiac transplantation.

3.4.6 Cardiac catheterisation

Since ischaemic heart disease is the commonest cause of chronic heart failure, some form of risk stratification and consideration for coronary revascularisation may be necessary. As well as determining the presence of coronary artery disease, cardiac catheterisation also allows further assessment of left-ventricular and valvular function. Right heart catheterisation assists in the determination of left-to-right shunting, pulmonary hypertension, pulmonary capillary wedge pressure, mitral-valve gradients, cardiac output and restricted ventricular filling. Occasionally, ventricular biopsy may be of benefit in patients with a cardiomyopathy of uncertain origin but rarely alters management as fibrosis and scarring are the end stage of many pathological processes.

3.4.7 Radionuclide ventriculography

Radionuclide ventriculography is particularly useful for the assessment of left-ventricular function in patients in whom a suitable echo window is difficult to achieve. It is better than echocardiography for the assessment of right-ventricular function but cardiac gating is required to improve image quality and, as such, is not suitable for patients with atrial fibrillation.

3.4.8 Cardiac magnetic resonance imaging

Cardiac magnetic resonance (CMR) imaging provides a comprehensive and reproducible analysis of cardiac anatomy and function. It allows the assessment of left and right-ventricular volume and mass (see Figure 3.3), global and regional function, myocardial thickness and

Figure 3.3 Patient with previous myocardial infarction, left-ventricular dilatation and wall thinning

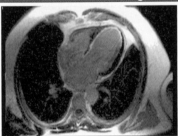

Cardiac magnetic resonance imaging showing anteroseptal myocardial infarction (revealed by late gadolinium enhancement) and associated left-ventricular dilatation and wall thinning. Four chamber view.

Figure 3.3 is reproduced with kind permission of Dr John Payne.

valvular anatomy. The pattern of late gadolinium enhancement may also provide clues to the aetiology of heart failure. For example, coronary artery disease is particularly associated with regional areas of subendocardial late enhancement, in contrast to the patchy, mid-wall pattern of enhancement often seen in association with dilated cardiomyopathy. CMR is particularly well suited for the investigation of patients with heart failure associated with congenital heart disease and can identify cardiac masses and pericardial disease. The application of CMR to a wide range of cardiac pathologies is currently the subject of intense research and its use is becoming relevant to a rapidly increasing range of conditions. It is, however, expensive and not readily available in all centres.

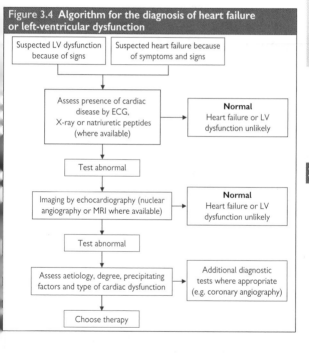

Figure 3.4 Algorithm for the diagnosis of heart failure or left-ventricular dysfunction

Figure 3.4 has been adapted from *Guidelines for the diagnosis and treatment of chronic heart failure: executive summary* (update 2005), with permission from the European Society of Cardiology and Oxford University Press.

Key references

Assomull, R., Pennell, D., Prasad, S. (2007). Cardiovascular magnetic resonance in the evaluation of heart failure. *Heart*, **93**, 985–92.

Battaglia, M., Pewsner, D., Juni, P., Egger, M., Bucher, H.C., Bachmann, L.M. Accuracy of B-type natriuretic peptide tests to exclude congestive heart failure: systematic review of test accuracy studies. *Arch. Intern. Med.*, **166**, 1073–80.

Hendel, R., Patel, M., Kramer, C., *et al.* (2006). ACCF/ACR/SCCT/SCMR/ASNC/NASCI/SCAI/SIR 2006 appropriateness criteria for cardiac computed tomography and cardiac magnetic resonance imaging: a report of the American College of Cardiology Foundation Quality Strategic Directions Committee Appropriateness Criteria Working Group, American College of Radiology, Society of Cardiovascular Computed Tomography, Society for Cardiovascular Magnetic Resonance, American Society of Nuclear Cardiology, North American Society for Cardiac Imaging, Society for Cardiovascular Angiography and Interventions, and Society of Interventional Radiology. *J. Am. Coll. Cardiol.*, **48**, 1475–97.

Hunt, S., Abraham, W., Chin, M., Feldman, A., Francis, G., Ganiats, T., *et al.* (2005). ACC/AHA 2005 Guideline Update for the Diagnosis and Management of Chronic Heart Failure in the Adult: a report of the American College of Cardiology/American Heart Association Task Force on Practice Guidelines *Circulation*, **112**, e154–235.

Kirkpatrick, J., Vannan, M., Narula, J., Lang, R. (2007). Echocardiography in heart failure: applications, utility, and new horizons. *J. Am. Coll. Cardiol.*, **50**, 381–96.

Scottish Intercollegiate Guidelines Network (SIGN). Management of chronic heart failure. Edinburgh: SIGN; 2007. (SIGN publication no. 95). Available from url: http://www.sign.ac.uk

Swedberg, K., Cleland, J., Dargie, H., *et al.* (2005). Guidelines for the diagnosis and treatment of chronic heart failure: executive summary (update 2005): The Task Force for the Diagnosis and Treatment of Chronic Heart Failure of the European Society of Cardiology. *Eur. Heart J.*, **26**, 1115–40.

White, J.A., Patel, M.R. (2007). The role of cardiovascular MRI in heart failure and the cardiomyopathies. *Cardiol Clin.*, **25**, 71–95.

Chapter 4

Assessment of prognosis in patients with chronic heart failure

Christopher Gale and Mark Kearney

Key Points

- The prognosis in patients with chronic heart failure is poor and worse than many malignancies.
- Patients frequently die from progressive heart failure or sudden death principally due to ventricular arrhythmia.
- The precise mechanisms for the modes of death from heart failure are unclear.
- Numerous potentially useful markers of prognosis exist.
- Assessment of prognosis may be determined non-invasively and when allied to physicians judgement may allow tailoring of therapies and aid discussions with patients and families regarding treatment strategies and life expectancy.

4.1 Introduction

Despite the use of state of the art therapies prognosis in patients with chronic heart failure (CHF) remains poor. In the last decade it has become increasingly appreciated that patients with CHF have two principal modes of death: sudden arrhythmic death, or progressive pump failure. Determining who is likely to suffer early mortality per se and patients destined to die suddenly or from progressive heart failure may allow the more accurate assessment of prognosis and help clinicians tailor therapies more appropriately.

4.2 All cause mortality in patients with chronic heart failure

The prognosis in patients with CHF is poor. Death rates in patients with controlled symptoms are >10% per year whereas life expectancy of patients with advanced CHF is even worse, typically 1–3 years (see Table 4.1).

There are data to suggest that CHF survival rates are as poor as those associated with many cancers. For example a Scotland-wide retrospective cohort study compared 5-year survival rates among individuals requiring a first admission to hospital in 1991 for heart failure, myocardial infarction, and the four most common types of cancer specific to men and women. For both men and women lung cancer was associated with the poorest unadjusted survival rate with a median survival time of 3–4 months. CHF was associated with the second poorest unadjusted survival rate with a median survival time of 16 months, only 25% of men and women survived to 5 years.

4.3 Mode of death

As discussed in Chapter 2, it is apparent that after an initial insult to the myocardium, patients suffer a gradual decline in myocardial function that may be interrupted by episodes of acute decompensation. A significant proportion of patients with stable CHF despite contemporary

Table 4.1 Large surveys of prognosis in chronic heart failure

Study	Number of patients	NYHA class	Mortality at year (%)					
			1	2	3	4	5	>5
Framingham (McKee, 1971)	219	I to IV	1	2	3	4	5	>5
Duke University (Califf, 1982)	236	I to III		26		58		70 (at 8 years)
Philadelphia and Minneapolis (Franciosa, 1983)	182	III to IV	20	30				
University of Pennsylvania (Wilson, 1983)	77	III to IV	34	59				
San Francisco and Montreal (Rockman, 1989)	238	III to IV	48	68				
Glasgow (Cleland, 1987)	152	II to IV	10	25	53	62	90	92 (at 7 years)
France (Komajda, 1990)	201	I to IV		41				
United Kingdom (Kearney, 2003)	553	I to III	4	7	10	13	20	47

NYHA = New York Heart Association.

therapies ultimately enter this vicious cycle of worsening left-ventricular function. Although many patients suffer a gradual decline in symptomatic status culminating in death due to cardiac decompensation it has become apparent that a large proportion of patients with CHF die suddenly. In the Framingham Study, the sudden death rate for patients with CHF was almost ten times the general age adjusted population rate. The mechanisms underlying progressive heart failure death and sudden death are not fully understood. If the mechanisms (and hence prognostic markers) underlying sudden death and death due to progressive CHF are different then therapeutic approaches needed to treat patients with CHF may need to be tailored for individual patients.

4.3.1 Mechanisms of progressive heart-failure death

As discussed in Chapter 2 the mechanisms underlying the progressive decline in left-ventricular systolic function characteristic of CHF are beginning to emerge. An initial insult to left-ventricular systolic performance stimulates the enhanced activity of a broad portfolio of compensatory systems, which have detrimental effects on cardiac function. Moreover left-ventricular dysfunction leads to perturbation of normal function of the lungs, kidneys, blood vessels, skeletal muscle, liver and possibly bone marrow. Some of these abnormalities can be quantified and offer prognostic information.

4.3.2 Mechanisms of sudden death

Sudden death in the context of CHF is typically interpreted to mean death due to sustained ventricular tachyarrhythmias, most often ventricular tachycardia degenerating into ventricular fibrillation. Sustained fatal ventricular arrhythmias are thought to require both a permissive substrate and a trigger (see Figure 4.1). A permissive substrate is a structural myocardial abnormality such as infarction, hypertrophy, dilatation, fibrosis, inflammation, or infiltration that results in either abnormal electrical activation or repolarization. Specific functional factors, including ischaemia, haemodynamic stress, and neurohumoral stimulation, act on this permissive substrate to convert the underlying structure into an unstable electrophysiological environment.

4.4 Predicting all-cause mortality in patients with CHF

A large number of prognostic variables may be measured in patients with CHF (see Table 4.2 for selected examples). These variables include but are not restricted to; abnormalities of cardiac size, shape, function and electrical activation, plasma measurements of renal function, neurohumoral activation, natriuretic peptides and inflammation, 12-lead and 24-hour ECG abnormalities, exercise capacity or changes in cardiac function during exercise. Patients with symptoms and signs at rest are easy to identify by clinical assessment. These patients have an annual mortality rate >25% even with optimal medical therapy, but they make up only a relatively small proportion of the CHF population. In ambulant patients with CHF it is more difficult to identify those at high risk of early death. The prognostic utility of different variables may be enhanced by using them in an integrated fashion in prognostic indices analogous to the staging systems used in many malignancies.

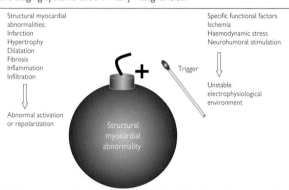

Figure 4.1 Mechanisms of sudden death in chronic heart failure. Sustained fatal ventricular arrhythmias require both a permissive substrate (structural myocardial abnormality) and a trigger (specific functional factors).

Table 4.2 Variables related to prognosis in chronic heart failure	
Severity of heart failure	NYHA class
	Exercise capacity (such as peak VO2)
Left-ventricular function	Heart size on chest X-ray
	Presence of third heart sound
	Left-ventricular ejection fraction
	Left-ventricular end-systolic volume
	Peak left-ventricular power output
Plasma markers	Sodium
	Creatinine
	Urate
	Brain natriuretic peptide
	High sensitivity C-reactive protein
	Magnesium
	Noradrenaline
ECG/24-hour Holter	Left bundle branch block
	Ventricular tachycardia
	Atrial fibrillation
	Left-ventricular hypertrophy
	Non-sustained ventricular tachycardia
	Heart rate variability
NYHA = New York Heart Association.	

4.5 **Prognostic indices**

A number of potentially useful models predicting mortality in different groups of patients with CHF have been published. The Seattle Heart Failure Model (Levy *et al.*) was derived from a cohort of 1125 ambulant heart-failure patients and validated in five additional cohorts. It used patients' demographics, medications, implantable-cardiac-defibrillator use, and laboratory results to predict survival at 1, 2, and 3 years.

A non-invasive risk model to identify patients with end-stage congestive heart failure suitable for transplant selection was derived by Aaronsen *et al.*, using data from 268 patients with advanced heart failure. However, most risk models have been derived from retrospective analyses or from populations entered into clinical trials of therapeutic agents where development of a predictive model was not the primary aim of the study. The United Kingdom Evaluation and Assessment of Risk Trial (UK-HEART) study developed prognostic indices in a highly character-ized group of patients that allowed the prediction of all cause mortality, sudden death, and death due to progressive CHF (see Table 4.3).

4.6 **Conclusion**

As our understanding of the pathophysiology of CHF has developed so have therapeutic approaches to its management. Despite these advances in therapy, some patients suffer from a rapid decline in

Table 4.3 Predictive variables for ambulant patients in the UK-HEART study	
Predictors of all cause mortality	Serum sodium
	Serum creatinine
	Left-ventricular end systolic diameter
	Electrocardiographic left-ventricular hypertrophy
	The standard deviation of each normal to normal RR interval over 24 hours (SDNN)
	Age
	Non-sustained ventricular tachycardia
Predictors of progressive heart failure death	Serum sodium
	Serum creatinine
	SDNN
Predictors of sudden death	Cardiothoracic ratio
	Non-sustained ventricular tachycardia on Holter
	QRS dispersion on 12 lead electro-cardiogram
	QT dispersion across leads V1–V6

left-ventricular function and die of decompensated CHF, whereas others maintain haemodynamic competence but suffer a fatal cardiac arrhythmia and die suddenly. Identifying patients at high risk per se and identifying patients at high risk of sudden death or progressive heart failure is an important aim as potential therapeutic strategies aimed at these processes may differ. Recent studies have demonstrated that it may be possible to identify patients at high risk of premature death and these different modes of death using non-invasive tests. However, at present these tests require validation and should be part of a global assessment of risk allied to clinician experience or intuition.

Key references

Kearney, M.T., Fox, K.A., Lee, A.J., et al. (2002). Predicting death due to progressive heart failure in patients with mild-to-moderate chronic heart failure. J. Am. Coll. Cardiol., **40**, 1801–8.

Lee, D.S., Austin, P.C., Rouleau, J.L., Liu, P.P., Naimark, D., Tu, J.V. (2003). Predicting mortality among patients hospitalized for heart failure: derivation and validation of a clinical model. JAMA, **290**, 2581–7.

Levy, W.C., Mozaffarian, D., Linker, D.T., et al. (2006). The Seattle Heart Failure Model: prediction of survival in heart failure. Circulation, **113**, 1424–33.

Lund, L.H., Aaronson, K.D., Mancini, D.M. (2003). Predicting survival in ambulatory patients with severe heart failure on beta-blocker therapy. Am. J. Cardiol., **92**, 1350–54.

Pocock, S.J., Wang, D., Pfeffer, M.A., et al. (2006). Predictors of mortality and morbidity in patients with chronic heart failure. Eur. Heart J., **27**, 65–75.

Aaronson, K.D., Schwartz, J.S., Chen, T.M., Wong, K.L., Goin, J.E., Mancini, D.M. (1997). Development and prospective validation of a clinical index to predict survival in ambulatory patients referred for cardiac transplant evaluation. Circulation, **95**, 2660–7.

Cowburn, P.J., Cleland, J.G. (2001). Endothelin antagonists for chronic heart failure: do they have a role? Eur. Heart J., **22**, 1772–84.

Chapter 5

Blockade of the renin–angiotensin–aldosterone system

Steven M. Shaw, John E. Macdonald
and Simon G. Williams

Key Points

- Blockade of the renin–angiotensin–aldosterone system is a cornerstone of treatment of patients with chronic heart failure (CHF).
- The use of angiotensin-converting enzyme (ACE) inhibitors in patients with CHF improves quality of life and prognosis across all stages of the disorder.
- The angiotensin receptor blockers are effective substitutes for ACE inhibitors.
- The combination of ACE inhibitors and angiotensin-receptor blockers is effective in reducing mortality and morbidity in patients with CHF.
- Spironolactone an aldosterone antagonist is effective in patients with more advanced heart failure; evidence in less severely symptomatic heart failure is awaited.

5.1 Background

As discussed in Chapter 2, excessive activation of the renin–angiotensin–aldosterone system (RAAS) has emerged as a key player in the pathophysiology of chronic heart failure (CHF). Targeting this maladaptive response has been a major advance in the treatment of CHF, improving prognosis and quality of life in large numbers of patients. This chapter discusses in more detail the physiology of this system and therapeutic approaches to blocking its detrimental actions.

5.2 **Physiology of the RAAS**

5.2.1 **Renin and angiotensin I**

The juxtaglomerular apparatus sited adjacent to the glomerulus of each nephron in the kidney is responsible for the production of the protease renin, in response to: 1) a reduction in sodium flux across the macula densa; 2) an increase in sympathetic nerve traffic to the juxtaglomerular apparatus; 3) a reduction in arteriolar transmural pressure; 4) An increase in circulating angiotensin II concentration.

When circulating blood volume is low, renin secretion increases via the above mechanisms. Upon release, renin cleaves angiotensinogen to produce angiotensin I, which is only weakly biologically active but is subsequently converted into the powerful vasoconstrictor angiotensin II, by the action of angiotensin-converting enzyme (ACE) (see Figure 5.1).

5.2.2 **Angiotensin II**

The lung is the main site of angiotensin II production. However, the heart, kidney, brain, and blood vessels also produce ACE and can synthesize angiotensin II from angiotensin I. Acting directly on the zona glomerulosa by binding to angiotensin II type-I receptors, angiotensin II primarily increases aldosterone secretion. In addition, it increases systemic vascular resistance by vasoconstriction, which subsequently increases blood pressure and hence cardiac afterload (see Chapter 2). Glomerular filtration rate and sodium delivery to the kidney are also reduced, thereby conserving sodium and increasing thirst.

Angiotensin II also induces necrosis and fibroblast proliferation in the myocardium. Furthermore, raised serum angiotensin II concentrations stimulate excessive adrenal production of aldosterone. Angiotensin II may also increase vascular and cardiac aldosterone synthesis, leading to the additional adverse effects caused by excessive aldosterone production.

5.2.3 **Aldosterone**

Aldosterone is the principal mineralocorticoid hormone, its main role is to preserve circulating volume. Within the kidney, it increases the permeability of the distal convoluted tubule and collecting duct allowing greater sodium and water resorption. This homoeostatic mechanism is usually appropriate, for example following haemorrhage. However, in CHF, detrimental secondary hyperaldosteronism occurs. Elevated aldosterone levels have a variety of detrimental effects in CHF, as shown in Figure 5.2.

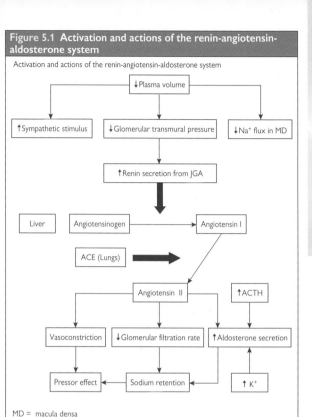

Figure 5.1 Activation and actions of the renin-angiotensin-aldosterone system

Activation and actions of the renin-angiotensin-aldosterone system

MD = macula densa

JGA = juxtaglomerular apparatus

ACE = angiotensin-converting enzyme

ACTH = adrenocorticotrophin

5.3 Pharmacological blockade of RAAS

5.3.1 ACE inhibitors

In the 1950s it was found that a peptide in snake venom inhibited the action of ACE and prevented the formation of angiotensin II. In 1975, Cushman and Ondetti produced the first oral ACE inhibitor (ACEI) captopril. Captopril possessed significant blood pressure lowering properties. In 1979 Turini and colleagues reported that an ACEI reduced preload and afterload, with a subsequent improvement of cardiac function when given to CHF patients. This finding led to the development of large randomized clinical trials, to evaluate whether ACEIs could improve survival in patients with CHF.

5.3.2 Key ACE inhibitor trials

One of the first mortality trials evaluating the use of ACEIs in CHF was the Cooperative North Scandinavian Enalapril Survival Study (CONSENSUS), which reported in 1987. In this randomized double-blinded trial, 253 patients with severe CHF—New York Heart Association (NYHA) class IV—were allocated to enalapril or placebo. After a mean follow up of 188 days, mortality was reduced in the enalapril arm by 40%.

The large Studies of Left-Ventricular Dysfunction (SOLVD) trial evaluated the use of Enalapril in patients with left-ventricular ejection fractions of less than 35%. Over a mean follow-up period of 41.4 months, 2569 patients were randomly assigned to take placebo or enalapril. A 16% relative-risk reduction of death resulted in the enalapril group with a 26% reduction of the combined secondary endpoint of hospitalization for heart failure and death. Shortly after, a series of similar trials ensued demonstrating favourable effects in patients with impaired left-ventricular function after myocardial infarction.

5.3.3 Angiotensin-receptor blockers

Despite the successful introduction of ACEIs, the reduction of circulating angiotensin II and aldosterone levels were variable and often incomplete in some patients with CHF. One potential mechanism accounting for this is the accumulation of angiotensin I. This substrate can then be converted to angiotensin II via non-ACE mechanisms. Angiotensin-receptor blockers were developed to directly antagonize the effect of angiotensin II on its receptor (AT1).

5.3.4 Key trials of angiotensin-receptor blockers

In 1997, the results of the first major study of angiotensin-receptor blockers in CHF (ELITE) were published. Treatment with losartan was compared with ACEI treatment with captopril in elderly patients. Patients were randomly assigned in a double-blind fashion to receive losartan or captopril and followed for 48 weeks. This study was designed primarily to demonstrate safety and efficacy advantages over ACEI. However, in *post hoc* analysis, a significant reduction in mortality was noted in the losartan group. Subsequently, the ELITE II trial was conducted to determine whether losartan was superior to captopril in reducing mortality from CHF. In 3152 patients, once daily losartan at a dose of 50 mg was compared with captopril 50 mg three-times daily. There was, however, no difference in the primary endpoint of all-cause mortality. It was concluded therefore that once daily dosing of 50 mg Losartan, was not superior in preventing death than standard ACE inhibition with captopril.

The Optimal Trial in Myocardial Infarction with Angiotensin II Antagonist Losartan compared losartan 50 mg once daily with captopril 50 mg three-times daily in patients after a myocardial infarction with CHF. After a mean follow up of 2.7 years there was no significant difference in the primary endpoint of all cause mortality despite a slight trend for benefit in the captopril arm.

The Valsartan in Heart Failure Trial (VaL-HeFT) later examined the effect of valsartan in patients with CHF, in addition to standard treatments, including ACEIs. Patients with NYHA class II-IV CHF were randomly assigned to receive 160 mg of valsartan or placebo twice daily for a mean duration of 23 months. No significant difference in mortality was seen between the two groups. However, there was a significant reduction in a combined endpoint of mortality and morbidity in the valsartan group primarily driven by a reduction in hospitalization for heart failure. In a subgroup analysis of patients who were not taking ACEIs, a large significant reduction in overall mortality was seen.

The CHARM trials programme evaluated the use of a newer angiotensin-receptor blocker candesartan in three discrete heart-failure populations:

- Patients with CHF and reduced left-ventricular systolic function already taking ACEIs (CHARM–added).
- Patients with CHF and reduced left-ventricular systolic function who were intolerant of ACE inhibitors (CHARM–alternative).
- Patients with CHF and preserved left-ventricular systolic function with ejection fraction greater than 40% (CHARM-preserved).

The CHARM-added study showed that the addition of candesartan to ACEI resulted in a significant reduction in cardiovascular death or admission to hospital for CHF. In addition, the secondary endpoint of cardiovascular death was also reduced. The CHARM–alternative study found that there was a significant reduction of the primary endpoint in the candesartan group, compared with placebo. Finally, in the CHARM–preserved study there was no statistical mortality benefit when candesartan was added to current treatment. However, hospital admissions for heart failure were reduced.

5.4 **Aldosterone antagonists**

5.4.1 **Spironolactone**

The steroid spironolactone, first synthesised in 1957, is a competitive antagonist of aldosterone and also reduces adrenocortical biosynthesis of aldosterone. It has been used clinically to treat Conn's syndrome, hypertension, ascites, nephritic syndrome, hirsuitism, and acne as well as CHF.

5.4.2 Trial of spironolactone in chronic heart failure

The Randomized Aldactone Evaluation Study (RALES) was an international, multicentre, double-blind trial reported in 1999. Patients were randomized to low-dose spironolactone (25–50 mg once daily) 1663 patients participated; the majority of whom were NYHA class III or IV. A significant 30% reduction in the primary endpoint of all cause mortality in the spironolactone arm resulted in the early cessation of the trial. A reduction in both sudden and progressive heart-failure death contributed to this finding. As a result spironolactone became a standard addition to pharmacological therapy for patients with moderate to severe CHF.

5.4.3 Eplerenone

Following the resurgence of interest in aldosterone blockade stimulated by the RALES trial, a new aldosterone blocker was introduced. Eplerenone is the first selective aldosterone-receptor antagonist. In contrast to spironolactone, it does not bind to oestrogen, progesterone, or androgen receptors. Therefore, the prevalence of gynaecomastia and impotence with eplerenone use is less than 1%.

5.4.4 The EPHESUS study

The Eplerenone Post-Acute Myocardial Infarction Heart Failure Efficacy and Survival Study (EPHESUS) was a large randomized, double-blind trial of eplerenone 25–50 mg daily compared with placebo for post myocardial infarction heart failure. Patients were followed up for a mean 16 months and were eligible for randomization 3–14 days after acute myocardial infarction if their left-ventricular ejection fraction was less than 40% and they had clinical signs of CHF. Death from any cause fell significantly. There was also a reduction in the combined endpoint of death from cardiovascular causes or hospitalization for cardiovascular events. Among the secondary endpoints significant reductions were seen in sudden cardiac death and hospitalization for heart failure.

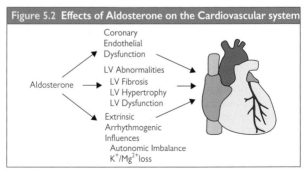

Figure 5.2 Effects of Aldosterone on the Cardiovascular system

Aldosterone

Coronary
Endothelial
Dysfunction

LV Abnormalities
LV Fibrosis
LV Hypertrophy
LV Dysfunction

Extrinsic
Arrhythmogenic
Influences
Autonomic Imbalance
K^+/Mg^{2+}loss

5.5 **Unanswered questions**

5.5.1 **What about aldosterone antagonists in less advanced heart failure?**

It is unknown whether the survival and morbidity benefits observed in RALES and EPHESUS extend to patients with mild symptoms or asymptomatic left-ventricular dysfunction. If similar benefits were seen in individuals with NYHA class I-II heart failure then treatment could be offered to these patients and the syndrome could be treated at an earlier stage. This is currently being evaluated in the Effect of Eplerenone in Chronic Systolic Heart Failure (EMPHASIZE-HF) trial, a long-term, placebo-controlled, outcomes trial. This trial is designed to include stable patients with NYHA functional class II chronic systolic heart failure randomized to eplerenone plus standard therapy or placebo plus standard therapy and followed up for up to 4 years.

5.6 **Conclusion**

Activation of the RAAS is central to the pathogenesis of CHF. The development of therapeutic strategies with ACE inhibitors, angiotensin receptor blockers, and aldosterone antagonists to attenuate elements of this system have reduced mortality and morbidity in patients across a range of classes of heart failure.

Key references

The CONSENSUS Trial Study Group (1987). Effects of enalapril on mortality in severe congestive heart failure. Results of the Cooperative North Scandinavian Enalapril Survival Study (CONSENSUS). *N. Engl. J. Med.*, **316**, 1429–35.

The SOLVD Investigators (1991). Effect of enalapril on survival in patients with reduced left-ventricular ejection fractions and congestive heart failure. *N. Engl. J. Med.*, **325**, 293–302.

Pfeffer, M.A., Braunwald, E., Moye, L.A., *et al.* (1992). Effect of captopril on mortality and morbidity in patients with left-ventricular dysfunction after myocardial infarction. Results of the survival and ventricular enlargement trial. The SAVE Investigators. *N. Engl. J. Med.*, **327**, 669–77.

Swedberg, K., Held, P., Kjekshus, J., Rasmussen, K., Ryden, L., Wedel, H. (1992). Effects of the early administration of enalapril on mortality in patients with acute myocardial infarction. Results of the Cooperative New Scandinavian Enalapril Survival Study II (CONSENSUS II). *N. Engl. J. Med.*, **327**, 678–84.

Effect of ramipril on mortality and morbidity of survivors of acute myocardial infarction with clinical evidence of heart failure. The Acute Infarction Ramipril Efficacy (AIRE) Study Investigators. *Lancet*, **342**, 821–28.

Pitt, B., Segal, R., Martinez, F.A., *et al.* (1997). Randomized trial of losartan versus captopril in patients over 65 with heart failure (Evaluation of Losartan in the Elderly Study, ELITE). *Lancet*, **349**, 747–52.

Pitt, B., Poole-Wilson, P.A., Segal, R., *et al.* (2000). Effect of losartan compared with captopril on mortality in patients with symptomatic heart failure: randomized trial--the Losartan Heart Failure Survival Study ELITE II. *Lancet*, **355**, 1582–7.

Pitt, B., Zannad, F., Remme, W.J., *et al.* (1999). The effect of spironolactone on morbidity and mortality in patients with severe heart failure. Randomized Aldactone Evaluation Study Investigators. *N. Engl. J. Med.*, **341**, 709–17.

Chapter 6

Beta-blockers and chronic heart failure

Edward Duncan and Marc Goethals

> ### Key Points
>
> - The combination of angiotensin-converting-enzyme inhibitors and beta-blockers is now established as the key therapy for patients with chronic heart failure (CHF) across all functional classes.
> - Beta-blockers may initially worsen symptoms but their long-term effects favourably influence key pathophysiological processes leading to death and disability in patients with CHF.
> - Beta-blockers have favourable effects on mortality from both progressive heart failure and sudden cardiac death.
> - A number of beta-blockers have been shown to be effective in randomized controlled clinical trials; these agents should be the treatment of choice in patients with CHF.
> - Airways disease is not a contraindication to beta-blockade; the benefits in most cases may outweigh the risks. The majority of such patients should undergo a trial of therapy.

6.1 Background

Beta-blockers are β-adrenoceptor antagonists that bind to these receptors resulting in a competitive and reversible antagonism of the effect of adrenergic stimulation. Historically beta-blockers have played an important role in the management of cardiovascular disease. These drugs were used for their antihypertensive, antianginal and antiarrhythmic properties. However, until relatively recently, beta-blockers were contraindicated in the setting of heart failure. In the late 1990s large double-blind randomized controlled trials clearly demonstrated that β-adrenoreceptor blockade is of significant benefit to patients with left-ventricular systolic dysfunction and heart failure. Beta-blockers are now recommended for routine use in heart failure in both American Heart Association and European Society of Cardiology guidelines.

6.2 **Rationale for use**

At rest, the normal human heart does not receive adrenergic support. Conversely the failing heart is adrenergically stimulated to maintain cardiac output in the short-term by increasing heart rate and contractility. As discussed in Chapter 2, it is now well established that this maladaptive process may ultimately be damaging to the failing heart.

Adrenergic stimulation unfavourably influences left-ventricular remodelling via a number of mechanisms. Besides promoting a larger infarct size after myocardial infarction, sympathetic drive promotes activation of the renin–angiotensin–aldosterone system, cardiac myocyte growth, and apoptosis. Norepinephrine is itself cardiotoxic causing apoptosis at the pathophysiological concentrations present in the failing heart.

There are three key adrenergic receptors in human cardiac myocytes: $\beta1$, $\beta2$, and $\alpha1$. Each receptor mediates a variety of potentially detrimental responses to adrenergic stimulation in the failing heart, including cardiac myocyte growth ($\beta1$, $\beta2$ + $\alpha1$), positive inotropic response ($\beta1$ + $\beta2$), positive chronotropic response ($\beta1$ + $\beta2$), myocyte toxicity ($\beta1$ + $\beta2$), and myocyte apoptosis ($\beta1$).

In what is thought to be a compensatory response, in the failing myocardium, $\beta1$ adrenoreceptor signalling is downregulated by a reduction in the $\beta1/\beta2$ receptor ratio from 70/30 to 60/40. Further downregulation of β-adrenoreceptor signal transduction downstream of the receptor results in a 50–60% reduction in total β-adrenoceptor signalling.

The rationale behind beta-blockade in the failing heart is that this may prove a therapeutic strategy that adds to the compensatory endogenous antiadrenergic response described above. Selective $\beta1$ blockade evolved to reduce peripheral $\beta2$-receptor mediated side effects, most notably bronchospasm. Beta-blockade has now been shown to have beneficial effects on many markers of ventricular remodelling (e.g. left-ventricular end-systolic volume and left-ventricular mass) and this has been translated into improved clinical outcomes. Notably, the combination of beta-blockers and angiotensin-converting-enzyme inhibitors has been shown to have a greater effect on cardiac function and mortality than either drug type used as monotherapy.

6.3 **Pharmacology**

6.3.1 **Classification**

Beta-blockers can be classified as either non-selective (those that produce competitive blockade of both β1 and β2 adrenoceptors) or β1 selective (those with greater affinity for the β1 than for the β2 receptor). However, selectivity is dose-dependent and diminishes at higher doses. Beta-blockers can be further classified by other properties. Some exert an agonist action both stimulating and blocking the β-adrenergic receptor, described as intrinsic sympathomimetic activity. Others cause peripheral vasodilatation via blockade of the α1-adrenoreceptor or stimulation of β2-adrenoreceptors. Finally, beta-blockers can be described as lipophilic or hydrophilic. Of the beta-blockers used in heart failure, metoprolol is approximately 75-fold β1 selective compared to β2 receptors. Bisoprolol is approximately 120-fold β1 selective. Carvedilol is only 7-fold β1 selective (less at high doses) and has potent α1-adrenoreceptor blocking properties resulting in moderate peripheral vasodilatation.

6.3.2 **Pharmacokinetic properties**

Lipophilic drugs (e.g. metoprolol) are readily absorbed when taken orally, but are extensively metabolised by the liver. They may accumulate in patients with reduced hepatic blood flow (e.g. elderly or congestive cardiac failure) but generally exhibit short elimination half-lives. These agents readily cross the blood–brain barrier. Hydrophilic drugs (atenolol) are less completely absorbed by the gastrointestinal tract and are excreted by the kidney. They have longer half-lives and barely cross the blood–brain barrier. Accumulation occurs if the glomerular filtration rate is reduced.

Of relevance to heart failure, bisoprolol has a low first pass metabolism, can cross the blood–brain barrier and is removed equally by renal and hepatic routes. Carvedilol has a high first-pass effect resulting in low oral bioavailability. It is cleared by the hepatic route.

6.3.3 **Mechanisms of action**

Beta-blockers improve cardiac function through the following mechanisms:

- Reduction of heart rate, prolongation of diastolic filling and coronary perfusion times
- Reduction of myocardial oxygen demand
- Improvement of myocardial energetics
- Reduction of myocardial oxidative stress
- Reduction of left-ventricular size and increase in ejection fraction

Beta-blockers are also antiarrhythmic and may prevent disease progression through antihypertensive and anti-ischaemic actions.

6.3.4 **Adverse effects of beta-blockers**

Beta-blockers are generally well tolerated but have a number of well-documented side effects. Cardiovascular side effects include bradycardia and hypotension, dizziness, and decreased peripheral blood flow—particularly in patients with peripheral vascular disease. Beta-blockers can also trigger a rise in airway resistance in patients with asthma or COPD with bronchospasm. Central side effects include fatigue, headache, insomnia, and sexual dysfunction. A meta-analysis of trials of beta-blockers suggests that the most significant side effects suffered by heart failure patients are hypotension, dizziness, and symptomatic bradycardia. However, fewer patients overall treated with beta-blockers withdrew from treatment than did treated with placebo.

6.3.5 **Contraindications**

Contraindications to the initiation of beta-blockers include severe asthma, symptomatic hypotension or bradycardia, and severe decompensated cardiac failure. Relative contraindications to their use include chronic obstructive lung disease without bronchospasm and significant peripheral vascular disease. The benefit such patients may receive from beta-blocker therapy may outweigh the risks. Diabetes and intermittent limb claudication are not absolute contraindications to the use of beta-blockers. The use of β1-selective agents may reduce the incidence of side effects in these patients.

6.3.6 **Dosing**

Appropriate dosing of beta-blockers varies with the clinical characteristics of the patient and the beta-blocker used. Generally beta-blockers should be started at a low dose and uptitrated slowly aiming to achieve target dose (bisoprolol 10 mg once daily, metoprolol controlled release/extended release (CR/XL) 200 mg once daily, carvedilol 50 mg twice daily) or the highest tolerated dose.

6.4 **Key trials of beta-blockers in heart failure**

The first important large randomized controlled trial was the Cardiac Insufficiency Bisoprolol Study (CIBIS I). Patients with New York Heart Association (NYHA) class III or IV heart failure and ejection fractions less than 40% were treated with bisoprolol or placebo. Bisoprolol significantly improved functional status but a trend to a reduction in mortality did not reach statistical significance. This was followed by CIBIS II; this was a multicentre, double-blind, placebo-controlled trial. Patients with NYHA class III or IV heart failure and ejection fractions less than 35% were treated with bisoprolol or placebo (in addition to angiotensin-converting-enzyme inhibitors and diuretics). CIBIS II was terminated early because of a significant mortality benefit of bisoprolol. Bisoprolol significantly reduced hospital admissions with worsening heart failure and all-cause mortality. Survival benefit was seen in those with both ischaemic and non-ischaemic left-ventricular dysfunction.

The Metoprolol CR/XL Randomized Intervention Trial in Congestive Heart Failure (MERIT-HF) study was a double-blind, randomized, placebo-controlled trial including 3991 patients with heart failure (NYHA class II-IV) and ejection fractions less than 40% treated with metoprolol CR/XL or placebo. Metoprolol was initiated at 12.5 mg or 25 mg once daily and uptitrated to 200 mg once daily over 8 weeks. As with CIBIS II, MERIT-HF was terminated early because of a significant mortality benefit of metoprolol. Metoprolol reduced both sudden death and deaths from worsening heart failure.

The Effect of Carvedilol on Survival in Severe Chronic Heart Failure (COPERNICUS) trial evaluated the effect of carvedilol on mortality in patients with advanced CHF. It was a randomized double-blind placebo controlled trial in which 2289 euvolaemic patients with NYHA class IV heart failure and ejection fractions less than 25% were randomized to receive either placebo or carvedilol (target dose 25 mg twice daily). COPERNICUS was terminated early because of a significant mortality benefit of carvedilol. Carvedilol significantly reduced all cause mortality, sudden cardiac death and rates of hospitalization with decompensated heart failure.

The comparison of carvedilol and metoprolol on clinical outcomes in patients with chronic heart failure in the Carvedilol or Metoprolol European Trial (COMET) did not unequivocally demonstrate a difference between metoprolol and carvedilol and the choice of agent therefore remains between metoprolol, bisoprolol, and carvedilol (see Table 6.1). It is important to note that in the majority of beta-blocker trials heart rate less than 55 bpm was an exclusion criteria, so there are no data on this type of patient with slow heart rate at commencement of beta-blockade.

Table 6.1 Key beta-blocker CHF trials

	NYHA II	NYHA III	NYHA IV
Metoprolol	MERIT-HF (41%)	MERIT-HF (55%)	MERIT-HF (4%)
Bisoprolol	–	CIBIS II (83%)	CIBIS II (17%)
Carvedilol	–	–	COPERNICUS (100%)
(%) = percentage of patients enrolled in each NYHA class			

6.5 **Current guidelines for beta-blocker use in patients with CHF**

The 2003 UK NICE guidelines for the management of CHF recommend that beta-blockers licensed for use in heart failure should be initiated in patients with heart failure due to left-ventricular dysfunction after diuretic and angiotensin-converting-enzyme-inhibitor therapy (where not contraindicated). The Amercian College of Cardiology–American Heart Association 2005 guidelines for the management of CHF in adults recommend use of beta-blockers in both stage B heart failure (structural abnormalities without symptoms) and stage C heart failure (structural abnormalities with current or previous symptoms of heart failure—see Figure 1.1 for details). The use of beta-blockers is also recommended in European Society of Cardiology guidelines for the management of CHF. The following practical guidelines are based on the European Society of Cardiology expert consensus document on beta-blockers 2004 (see Box 6.1 and Table 6.2).

Box 6.1 Prescribing beta-blockers

Who should receive a beta-blocker?
All patients with CHF and systolic dysfunction where beta-blockers not contraindicated.

What to promise?
Beta-blockers improve prognosis and reduce hospitalizations, some patients report symptom reduction.

When to start?
In stable patients without evidence of fluid overload, start angiotensin-converting-enzyme inhibitors first unless contraindicated NYHA class IV patients should be referred for specialist advice.

Dose?
Start with a low dose and increase slowly, consider doubling dose every 2 weeks; aim for target dose or highest tolerated dose (see Table 6.2).

Table 6.2 Dosing strategy for beta-blockers in patients with CHF

Beta-blocker	Starting dose (mg)	Target dose (mg)
Bisoprolol	1.25 once daily	10 once daily
Carvedilol	3.125 twice daily	25–50 twice daily
Metoprolol CR/XL	12.5–25 once daily	200 once daily

6.5.1 **Monitoring**

Monitor for heart failure symptoms, fluid retention or weight gain, hypotension, and bradycardia.

6.5.2 **Problem solving**

The natural history of heart failure means that beta-blockers may need to be reduced or discontinued at times if other measures to manage symptoms fail. Always consider reintroducing beta-blockers and up titrating when patients become stable. Seek specialist advice when unsure.

1. Symptomatic hypotension (dizziness, light headedness):
   Re-consider need for other medications e.g. calcium channel blockers, nitrates. Consider reduction of diuretic dose if no evidence of congestion.
2. Worsening symptoms and signs of heart failure (breathlessness, oedema, weight gain, fatigue): Increase dose of diuretic with or without angiotensin-converting-enzyme inhibitor. Consider reducing dose of beta-blockers, especially if no response to increased diuretic. Look for cause of deterioration.
3. Bradycardia: Assess symptoms. Perform electrocardiogram to exclude heart block. Review need for other heart-rate lowering drugs (digoxin, amiodarone, diltiazem). Consider reducing beta-blockers dose. Consider pacemaker.
4. Severe decompensated heart failure (heart failure, pulmonary oedema, shock): Admit patient to hospital. Consider discontinuation of beta-blockers.

6.6 **Conclusions**

Beta-blockers should be considered and commenced if possible in all patients with CHF. An initial deterioration in symptoms may occur that can often be dealt with by increasing the dose of loop diuretic the patient is taking. A number of beta-blockers have been shown to be effective in randomized controlled trials and these agents should be used ahead of non-evidence based therapies.

Key references

CIBIS Investigators and Committees (1994). A randomized trial of beta-blockade in heart failure. The Cardiac Insufficiency Bisoprolol Study (CIBIS). *Circulation*, **90**, 1765–73.

CIBIS Investigators and Committees (1999). Cardiac Insufficiency Bisoprolol Study (CIBIS II). *Lancet*, **353**, 9–13.

Metoprolol CR/XL (1999). Randomized Intervention Trial in Congestive Heart Failure (MERIT-HF). *Lancet*, **353**, 2001–6.

For the carvedilol prospective randomized cumulative survival study group (2001). Effect of carvedilol on survival in severe chronic heart failure (COPERNICUS). *N. Engl. J. Med.*, **344**, 1651–8.

Comparison of carvedilol and metoprolol on clinical outcomes in patients with chronic heart failure in the carvedilol or metoprolol european trial (COMET). *Lancet*, **362**, 7–13.

Chapter 7

Device therapy

Khaled Albouaini and D. Justin Wright

Key Points

- Conduction defects are common in patients with chronic heart failure, and are a marker of adverse prognosis.
- The mechanical ventricular dys-synchrony associated with conduction defects is now a target for therapeutic intervention in some patients with chronic heart failure (CHF).
- Resynchronization with biventricular pacemakers has been shown to improve mortality and quality of life in selected patients with CHF.
- Ventricular arrhythmia is a common cause of death in patients with CHF.
- Implantable cardioverter defibrillators improve prognosis in selected patients with CHF.

7.1 Cardiac resynchronization therapy

7.1.1 Background

One quarter to one third of patients with chronic heart failure (CHF) have left-bundle branch block or other conduction defects manifest by abnormalities of the QRS complex on the 12-lead electrocardiogram. Conduction abnormalities are associated with abnormal contraction of the left ventricle; this electromechanical dys-synchrony has been shown to exacerbate pre-existing cardiac dysfunction and has recently emerged as an attractive therapeutic target.

7.1.2 Rationale for cardiac resynchronization therapy

Cardiac pacing as a potential therapy for CHF was first described in 1994 by Cazeau et al. and Bakker et al. in patients with severe drug-refractory heart failure without conventional pacemaker indications. The aim was to stimulate the right and left ventricles to contract simultaneously and therefore augment cardiac output. This process is referred to as cardiac resynchronization therapy (CRT).

7.1.3 CRT implantation technique

Two main approaches are used to achieve left-ventricular pacing. The transvenous approach is the most commonly used and requires catheter cannulation of the coronary sinus to allow delivery of a pacing lead into the epicardial vein serving the left-ventricular free wall (see Figure 7.1 and Figure 7.2). The second is a surgical approach, which tends to be used when the transvenous approach fails, and is performed by placement of the left-ventricular lead under direct vision via thoracotomy or thoracoscopy.

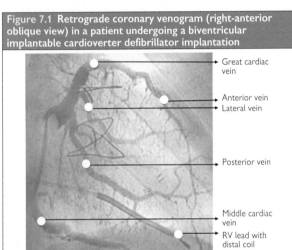

Figure 7.1 Retrograde coronary venogram (right-anterior oblique view) in a patient undergoing a biventricular implantable cardioverter defibrillator implantation

- Great cardiac vein
- Anterior vein
- Lateral vein
- Posterior vein
- Middle cardiac vein
- RV lead with distal coil

Figure 7.2 Chest radiograph shows a left-sided biventricular pacemaker with three leads: right-atrial lead, left-ventricular lead, and right-ventricular lead

- Pulse generator
- RA lead
- LV lead through the coronary sinus
- RV lead

7.1.4 **CRT clinical trials**

Several studies in the mid-1990s reported the acute haemodynamic benefits of biventricular pacing including reduction of left-ventricular filling pressure and severity of mitral regurgitation, as well as an improvement in ejection fraction and cardiac index. These benefits prompted several other studies to examine the short-term effects of biventricular pacing in patients with severe heart failure and electrical dys-synchrony. These studies demonstrated improved quality of life and clinical status.

Large randomized clinical trials have demonstrated the long-term benefits of CRT. COMPANION (Comparison of Medical Therapy, Pacing and Defibrillation in Heart Failure) was a randomized controlled study in which patients with New York Heart Association (NYHA) functional class III or IV heart failure, ejection fractions less than 35%, and QRS duration of 120 ms or more were randomly allocated to receive optimal medical therapy alone or in combination with CRT pacing (CRTP) or with CRT and implantable cardioverter defibrillator (CRTD). The risk of death or hospitalization for heart failure was reduced by 34% in the CRTP group and by 40% in the CRTD. CRTP insignificantly reduced the risk of the secondary endpoint of death from any cause by 24%, while CRTD significantly reduced this risk by 36%. Equal benefits were noted both in patients with ischaemic and nonischaemic aetiologies of heart failure.

In the CARE-HF study (Cardiac Resynchronization in Heart Failure), patients with predominantly NYHA functional class III symptoms were randomized to receive optimal medical therapy alone or with CRT. Patients were eligible if they were in sinus rhythm, had ejection fractions less than 35%, QRS duration greater than 150 ms or QRS duration between 120 ms and 150 ms and two of three echocardiography criteria for dys-synchrony. The primary endpoint was the time to death or unplanned hospitalization for a major cardiovascular event. After a mean follow-up of 29.4 months, the primary endpoint was reached in 39% of patients in CRT group compared with 55% on control medical therapy. This was the first study to show benefit for CRT with respect to survival as a single endpoint.

COMPANION and CARE-HF provide compelling evidence that CRT, with or without implantable cardioverter defibrillator (ICD), reduces mortality and hospitalization from heart failure. The benefit of CRT-ICD therapy was demonstrated by the observation that in the COMPANION trial, 36% of the deaths in the CRTP arm were sudden, very similar to the 35% in CARE-HF. The absence of ICD back up in both studies showed that despite the benefits of CRT pacing therapy, one-third of the fatalities were due to sudden death. The CRTD arm of COMPANION reduced the sudden-cardiac-death incidence to 16%. In terms of absolute mortality, 7% of patients in the

CRT limb of CARE-HF died suddenly, compared with only 2.9% in the CRTD limb of COMPANION.

7.1.5 Patient selection for CRT

Cardiac resynchronization therapy is recommended by the UK National Institute of Health and Clinical Excellence (NICE; technology appraisal guidance 120 issued in May 2007) in patients with heart failure who fulfil the following criteria:

- They are currently experiencing or have recently experienced NYHA class III–IV symptoms.
- They are in sinus rhythm:
  - either with a QRS duration of 150 ms or longer estimated by standard electrocardiogram
  - or with a QRS duration of 120–149 ms estimated by electrocardiogram and mechanical dys-synchrony that is confirmed by echocardiography.
- They have a left-ventricular ejection fraction of 35% or less.
- They are receiving optimal pharmacological therapy.

The UK NICE guidelines do not cover patients in atrial fibrillation; however, substudies (MUSTIC and CARE-HF) revealed maintained benefit from CRT in patients who either have atrial fibrillation at recruitment or develop it during the follow up.

Identifying patients with significant ventricular dys-synchrony is important, as they are most likely to respond to CRT. QRS duration determined from the surface electrocardiogram is the most commonly used predictor. All subgroup analyses show the greatest benefit from CRT in patients with QRS of 150 ms or more. However, if the current selection criteria are used (QRS duration greater than 120 ms), 20–30% of patients fail to respond clinically. This may be due to the fact that ventricular dys-synchrony is not always predicted by an electrocardiogram with QRS duration greater than 120 ms or the fact that a normal QRS duration could be compatible with significant mechanical dys-synchrony. Therefore to identify potential responders for CRT, both QRS duration and cardiac synchronicity should ideally be assessed. Post-implant follow-up is also important to evaluate the clinical response and ensure the optimal function of the device. This is usually done by assessing the clinical state of the patient as well as echocardiography to assess improvements in left-ventricular size, shape, and function. Device interrogation is performed to ensure maximal use of biventricular pacing mode (>90–95% of the time) and echocardiography can be used further for optimisation.

7.2 **Implantable cardioverter defibrillators and CHF**

7.2.1 **Sudden cardiac death in patients with CHF**

As discussed in Chapter 4, sudden death is a frequent mode of death in patients with CHF and the majority of sudden cardiac deaths are due to ventricular tachyarrhythmias. Prevention of sudden cardiac deaths can be primary, defined as prevention of a first life-threatening arrhythmic event, or secondary, which refers to the prevention of an additional life-threatening event in survivors of sudden cardiac events.

7.2.2 **Evolution of implantable-cardioverter-defibrillator therapy**

The first successful implantation of an implantable cardioverter defibrillator occurred in the late 1970s. Over the last three decades, the implantable cardioverter defibrillator has undergone a remark-able transformation in both size and capability. Early devices were large and required thoracotomy and implantation in the abdomen. The pulse generator had a life of less than 2 years, had almost no diagnostic capabilities, and had pacing capabilities that were limited only to backup ventricular pacing. Current devices are capable of delivering antitachycardia pacing, low energy cardioversion, and high-energy defibrillation therapy. They have also the capability to store the morphology and rates of arrhythmias before, during, and after therapy, with a longevity approaching 5 years.

7.2.3 **Benefits of implantable cardioverter defibrillators in patients with CHF: clinical trials**

Initially, implantable cardioverter defibrillators were only considered in patients who had survived a cardiac arrest or an episode of sus-tained ventricular tachycardia that was refractory to drug therapy. However, the results of clinical trials over the past decade have established their use as a cornerstone of therapy for all patients at high risk for sudden cardiac death. Currently, the majority of new implants are performed on primary prevention grounds. The details of the key studies involving patients with heart failure or left-ventricular dysfunction can be found in Table 7.1.

7.2.4 **UK NICE guidelines**

Implantable cardioverter defibrillators are recommended by the NICE (technology appraisal guidance 95, issued in January 2006) for patients in the following categories.

Table 7.1 Clinical trials of implantable cardioverter defibrillators for heart failure or left-ventricular dysfunction alone

Trial (Year)	Inclusion criteria	N	Comparison	Primary endpoint	Main finding	Number needed to treat (36 months)
Second Multicenter Automatic Defibrillator Implantation Trial (MADIT-II), 2002	NYHA I–III, EF ≤30%, remote MI (>1 month)	1232	ICD vs. best medical therapy	All-cause mortality	31% relative reduction in primary endpoint (P = 0.02) with ICD	10
Amiodarone Versus Implantable Cardio-verter Defibrillator Trial (AMIOVIRT), 2003	NYHA I–IV, EF ≤35%, dilated cardiomyopathy, NSVT	103	ICD vs. best medical therapy	All-cause mortality	No significant alteration (P = 0.8) with ICD	39
Cardiomyopathy Trial (CAT), 2002	NYHA II–III, EF ≤30%, dilated cardiomyopathy, recent onset heat failure (≤9 months)	104	ICD vs. best medical therapy	All-cause mortality	No significant alteration (P = 0.6) with ICD	12

Table 7.1 (Contd.)

Comparison of Medical Therapy, Pacing, and Defibrillation in Heart failure (COMPANION), 2004	NYHA III–IV, EF ≤35%, nonrecent MI or CABG (≥days), QRS ≥120 ms, PR ≥150 ms, recent heart failure hospitalization (<12 months), and non-recent onset of heart failure (>6 months)	903	Resynchronization ICD vs. best medical therapy	All-cause mortality or hospitalization	20% relative risk reduction in primary endpoint (P = 0.01) with resynchronization ICD	5
Sudden Cardiac Death Heart Failure Trial (SCD-HeFT), 2005	NYHA II–III, EF ≤35%, no recent MI or revascularization (>30 days), non-recent heart failure onset (>3 months)	1676	ICD vs. placebo	All-cause mortality	23% relative reduction in primary endpoint (P<0.01) with ICD	23
Defibrillators in Non-Ischaemic Cardiomyopathy Treatment Evaluation (DEFINITE), 2005	NYHA I–III, EF ≤35%, dilated cardiomyopathy, NSVT, or ≥10 PVCs/hour	458	ICD vs. best medical therapy	All-cause mortality	35% relative reduction in primary endpoint (P = 0.08) with ICD	24

CABG = coronary artery bypass graft; EF = ejection fraction; ICD = implantable cardioverter defibrillator; MI = myocardial infarction; NSVT = non-sustained ventricular tachycardia; NYHA = New York Heart Association functional class; PVC = premature ventricular complex.

Secondary prevention, that is, for patients who present, in the absence of a treatable cause, with one of the following

- having survived a cardiac arrest due to either ventricular tachycardia or ventricular fibrillation
- spontaneous sustained ventricular tachycardia causing syncope or significant haemodynamic compromise
- sustained ventricular tachycardia without syncope or cardiac arrest, and who have an associated reduction in ejection fraction (left-ventricular ejection fraction of less than 35%) (no worse than NYHA class III).

Primary prevention, that is, for patients who have the following

1. A history of previous (more than 4 weeks) myocardial infarction and: either
   a) left-ventricular dysfunction with an left-ventricular ejection fraction of less than 35% (no worse than class NYHA III), and
   b) non-sustained ventricular tachycardia on Holter (24-hour electrocardiogram) monitoring, and
   c) inducible ventricular tachycardia on electrophysiological testing
   or
   d) left-ventricular dysfunction with an left-ventricular ejection fraction of less than 30% (no worse than NYHA class III) and
   e) QRS duration of equal to or more than 120 ms
2. A familial cardiac condition with a high risk of sudden death, including long QT syndrome, hypertrophic cardiomyopathy, Brugada syndrome or arrhythmogenic right-ventricular dysplasia, or undergone surgical repair of congenital heart disease.

7.3 Conclusions

Device therapy over the last decade has emerged as an important treatment option in patients with CHF. Whilst selection of patients who will definitely derive benefit from both CRT and ICD remains a challenge, given to the right patients these devices have the potential to improve quality of life and prognosis.

Key references

Linde, C., Leclerc, C., Rex, S., *et al.* (2002). Long-term benefit of biventricular pacing in congestive heart failure: Results from the Multisite Stimulation in Cardiomyopathy (MUSTIC) Study. *J. Am. Coll. Cardiol.*, **40**, 111–8.

Young, J.B., Abraham, W.T., Smith, A.L., *et al.* (2003). Combined cardiac resynchronization and implantable cardioversion defibrillation in advanced chronic heart failure: the MIRACLE ICD trial. *JAMA*, **289**, 2685–94.

Cleland, J.G.F., Daubert, J.C., Erdmann, E., *et al.* for the Cardiac Resynchronization in Heart Failure study (CARE-HF) Study investigators (2005). The effect of cardiac resynchronization on morbidity and mortality in heart failure. *N. Engl. J. Med.*, **352**, 1539–49.

Moss, A.J., Hall, W.J., Cannom, D.S., *et al.* (2002). Improved survival with an implanted defibrillator in patients with coronary disease at high risk for ventricular arrhythmia. *N. Engl. J. Med.*, **335**, 1933–40.

Bansch, D., Antz, M., Boczor, S., *et al.* (2002). Primary prevention of sudden cardiac death in idiopathic dilated cardiomyopathy: The Cardiomyopathy Trial (CAT). *Circulation*, **105**, 1453–8.

Strickberger, S.A., Hummel, J.D., Bartlett, T.G., *et al.* (2003). Amiodarone versus implantable cardioverter-defibrillator: randomized trial in patients with nonischaemic dilated cardiomyopathy and asymptomatic nonsustained ventricular tachycardia-AMIOVIRT. *J. Am. Coll. Cardiol.*, **41**, 1707–12.

Kadish A, Dyer A, Daubert JP, *et al.* (2004). Prophylactic defibrillator implantation in patients with nonischaemic dilated cardiomyopathy. *N. Engl. J. Med.*, **350**, 2151–8.

Moss, A.J., Zareba, W., Hall, W.J., *et al.* (2002). Prophylactic implantation of a defibrillator in patients with myocardial infarction and reduced ejection fraction. *N. Engl. J. Med.*, **346**, 877–83.

Bardy, G.H., Lee, K.L., Mark, D.B., et al. (2005). Amiodarone or an implantable cardioverter-defibrillator for congestive heart failure. *N. Engl. J. Med.*, **352**, 225–37.

Chapter 8

Inherited cardiomyopathies

Carey Edwards and Sanjay Sharma

Key Points

- Inherited cardiomyopathies are a diverse group of genetically determined diseases of the heart muscle that may lead to heart failure or sudden cardiac death.
- Awareness of inherited cardiomyopathies enables early diagnosis, appropriate risk stratification and prevention of sudden death in young individuals and their relatives.
- Hypertrophic cardiomyopathy is the most common cardiomyopathy affecting one in 500 people and exhibits marked heterogeneity in terms of its natural history, clinical presentation and cardiac morphology.
- Arrhythmogenic right-ventricular cardiomyopathy is a relatively novel inherited cardiomyopathy and is the leading cause of sudden death during sport in young athletes in Italy.
- The diagnosis of arrhythmogenic right-ventricular cardiomyopathy can be challenging as many individuals are asymptomatic or express minimal symptoms and the diagnosis relies on several electrocardiographic and cardiac imaging modalities.

8.1 Background

Whilst ischaemic heart disease and hypertension account for the vast majority of disease, inherited primary heart-muscle disorders and hereditary systemic diseases affecting heart muscle are important causes particularly in the young. In this chapter, we consider inherited forms of cardiomyopathy under the headings hypertrophic cardiomyopathy (HCM), arrhythmogenic right-ventricular cardiomyopathy (ARVC), familial dilated cardiomyopathy (DCM), infiltrative cardiomyopathies, and left-ventricular non-compaction (LVNC).

8.2 Hypertrophic cardiomyopathy

HCM is defined by left-ventricular hypertrophy in the absence of a cardiac cause or moderate-severe hypertension. It is inherited as an autosomal dominant trait and affects people of all ages, sexes, and ethnic origins. The prevalence of HCM in the general population is one in 500.

8.2.1 Aetiology

Mutations in genes encoding sarcomeric contractile proteins are responsible for 60–70% of cases of HCM. The most common mutations implicated affect cardiac β-myosin heavy chain, troponin T, and cardiac myosin binding protein C, which account for 90% of all HCM due to sarcomeric protein disease.

Over 150 mutations have been identified in ten sarcomeric contractile proteins (see Table 8.1). The morphology, clinical presentation, and prognosis may be determined by the genotype. Mutations of the gene encoding troponin T are generally associated with only mild hypertrophy but also an increased risk in sudden death, whilst mutations in cardiac myosin binding protein C exhibit age related penetrance and late-onset disease.

8.2.2 Pathology

Macroscopically HCM may affect both ventricles. Hypertrophy is usually asymmetrical most commonly involving the interventricular septum and left-ventricular free wall to a greater extent than the posterior wall; however, almost any pattern of left-ventricular hypertrophy is possible. Structural abnormalities of the mitral valve occur including increased leaflet area. Elongation of the mitral valve leaflets and malposition or anomalous insertion of the papillary muscles are recognised features of HCM and are partly responsible for dynamic left-ventricular outflow tract obstruction.

Table 8.1 Contractile proteins affected by disease causing mutations in HCM	
Protein	% cases
Cardiac β-myosin heavy chain	30–40
Cardiac troponin T	10–20
Cardiac myosin binding protein C	20–30
α-tropomyosin	5
Cardiac troponin I	5
Essential myosin light chain	<5
Regulatory myosin light chain	<5
Cardiac actin	<5
Titin	<5

The histological hallmark of HCM is patchy myocyte disarray and interstitial fibrosis. Myocardial cells are hypertrophied and often bizarre in shape. These findings are not specific to hypertrophic cardiomyopathy; however, the extent of disarray is far greater in subjects with HCM.

8.2.3 **Pathophysiology**

Diastolic dysfunction

Left-ventricular hypertrophy is associated with impaired myocardial relaxation. Consequently left-ventricular end diastolic and left atrial pressures become raised leading to pulmonary venous congestion.

Obstruction

Approximately 25% of patients have evidence of left-ventricular outflow-tract obstruction at rest. The mechanisms leading to outflow obstruction are complex. The combination of hyperdynamic left-ventricular contraction, septal hypertrophy, narrow left-ventricular outflow tract, elongated mitral valve leaflets, and malposition of papillary muscles causes systolic anterior motion of the anterior mitral valve leaflet through Venturi forces. The resulting septal-mitral valve leaflet contact impedes left-ventricular ejection.

Ischaemia

Patients with HCM may present with typical angina even with normal coronary arteries. This may be explained by the oxygen requirements of the hypertrophied muscle exceeding coronary supply. Other factors thought to be involved include raised diastolic pressures preventing diastolic coronary artery flow and the disarrayed structure of the hypertrophied muscle results in inefficient contraction.

8.2.4 **Clinical features**

HCM exhibits marked heterogeneity in terms of cardiac morphology, clinical presentation, and natural history. Presentation may be at any age. The majority of patients remain asymptomatic or experience minimal symptoms. Adults are more likely to present with symptoms though 50% of patients are diagnosed incidentally on routine health checks or through family screening of affected individuals. The cardinal symptoms of HCM include chest pain, dyspnoea, palpitation and syncope. Unfortunately, sudden cardiac death may be the first presentation particularly in adolescent individuals, young adults and athletes aged less than 35 years.

8.2.5 **Investigating patients with suspected or diagnosed HCM**

Electrocardiography

There are no specific electrocardiographic changes unique to HCM though 12-lead electrocardiography remains a sensitive test, with 95–98%

patients with HCM having an abnormal test. Electrocardiographic changes usually precede the onset of left-ventricular hypertrophy and in the context of familial disease, are an early marker of the disorder in affected children.

Characteristic electrocardiographic changes include ST segment and T wave abnormalities, specifically T wave inversions, large magnitude QRS complexes, Romhilt-Estes points score of 5 for left-ventricular hypertrophy, pathological Q-waves and left bundle branch block (see Figure 8.1). Deep T-wave inversions in the anterior and inferior leads are a recognized manifestation of apical HCM. Isolated Sokolow-Lyon voltage criterion for left-ventricular hypertrophy is not a characteristic electrocardiographic feature of hypertrophic cardiomyopathy.

Imaging

Echocardiography is currently the gold-standard investigation in the diagnosis of HCM and is useful in demonstrating the pattern and magnitude of left-ventricular hypertrophy. The identification of left-ventricular hypertrophy greater than 15 mm is highly suggestive of the diagnosis; however, milder hypertrophy is diagnostic in the context of a family history of HCM. Left-ventricular hypertrophy may not become manifest until the pubertal growth spurt.

Other characteristic features of the disorder include a small left-ventricular cavity size, increased left-atrial diameter, hyperdynamic systolic function, left-ventricular outflow obstruction due to SAM and impaired diastolic function. Doppler echocardiography is used to quantify left-ventricular outflow tract obstruction.

Figure 8.1 An electrocardiogram showing giant T-wave inversion suggestive of apical HCM

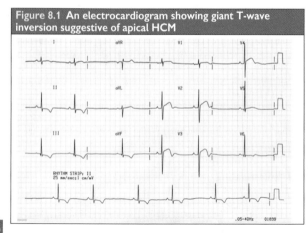

Cardiac magnetic resonance imaging is increasingly used in the assessment of patients with HCM and is particularly useful in the diagnosis of apical HCM and assessment of the left-ventricular free wall.

Cardiac catheterisation
Cardiac catheterisation has no role in the diagnosis of HCM. Coronary angiography may be necessary to exclude coexisting coronary artery disease in middle-aged patients with angina.

Cardiopulmonary exercise testing
Exercise testing is useful in the quantification of functional capacity through measurement of the peak oxygen consumption (pVO_2) and in risk stratification. Almost 25% of patients with HCM exhibit an abnormal blood pressure response to exercise (i.e. failure of systolic blood pressure to increase by 20 mm Hg from rest to peak exercise). An abnormal blood pressure response to exercise is a risk marker for sudden cardiac death.

24–48 hour Holter monitor
24–48 hour Holter monitoring identifies individuals with sustained or non-sustained ventricular tachycardia, another risk marker for sudden cardiac death particularly in young patients.

Genetic testing
Genetic testing is not routinely used in the diagnosis of HCM and continues to remain a research tool. The genetic heterogeneity of the disease makes genetic testing labour intensive, time consuming, and expensive. Mutations are identified in only 60% of patients and the diagnosis may not be available for up to 12 months. However, the identification of a causal genetic mutation enables cascade screening and enables early diagnosis prior to the development of left-ventricular hypertrophy.

8.2.6 Management of HCM
The aim of management is to improve symptoms, relieve left-ventricular outflow tract obstruction and prevent arrhythmias and sudden cardiac death.

Lifestyle modification
The strong association between sudden death and exercise in HCM makes it prudent to advise all affected individuals to abstain from all high-dynamic and high-intensity sports.

Symptomatic treatment
Beta-blockers and Ca^{2+} antagonists are the mainstay of symptomatic treatment. Their negative chronotropic effect prolongs diastolic filling. Beta-blockers are used as first-line therapy in patients with left-ventricular outflow obstruction as vasodilatation caused by Ca^{2+}

channel antagonists can worsen outflow tract obstruction and precipitate severe pulmonary oedema.

There is no evidence that treatment slows the progression of disease. Thus medical therapy should not be instituted in asymptomatic patients with the exception of patients with massive hypertrophy or evidence of outflow tract obstruction.

In about 5% of patients chronic ischaemia and ongoing myocardial fibrosis is associated with progressive myocardial thinning, left-ventricular dilatation and systolic impairment. In this group standard heart-failure treatment utilizing diuretic, angiotensin-converting-enzyme inhibitors and beta-blockers ameliorates symptoms.

Obstruction

The three main modalities used to treat left-ventricular outflow obstruction include pharmacotherapy; alcohol induced septal ablation and surgical myomectomy.

Beta-blockers are the mainstay of pharmacological therapy but disopyramide may be added to symptomatic patients with persisting severe (>60 mm Hg) outflow gradients. Both drugs are effective through their negative inotropic effects on the left ventricle, which reduces systolic anterior motion. Disopyramide should not be used alone as it has the potential to shorten atrioventricular node-conduction time, which may be problematic in patients with rapid paroxysms of atrial fibrillation.

Alcohol ablation of the hypertrophied septum is a relatively new technique with satisfactory symptomatic and haemodynamic results. Alcohol is injected into the first septal artery inducing a controlled myocardial infarction. The technique carries a 10–30% risk of complete heart block requiring permanent pacing. The long-term risks of heart failure and scar-related arrhythmias remain unknown.

Left-ventricular outflow obstruction can be abolished by surgical septal myomectomy. The operation relieves obstruction in 90% of patients and has been shown to relieve symptoms in 70% of patients for 5 years or more. The surgical mortality is relatively high and may exceed 10% in inexperienced hands.

Cardiac pacing has been used to induce dys-synchrony in an attempt to reduce outflow-tract gradients. Symptomatic relief described in early trials appears to be largely due to placebo effect. Pacing remains a therapeutic option in elderly patients unsuitable for definitive treatment of obstruction in which medical therapy has failed.

Arrhythmias

Supraventricular arrhythmias are treated with amiodarone. Patients with atrial fibrillation should be anticoagulated to reduce the risk of systemic thromboembolism, a recognized cause of morbidity in HCM. The management of ventricular tachycardia is described below.

8.2.7 Risk stratification of patients

The annual mortality from HCM is relatively low being 0.5–1% in the adult population and 3–5% in children and adolescents. Identification of the subgroup of patients with HCM at high risk of sudden death remains challenging.

Patients who have survived a cardiac arrest or have sustained ventricular tachycardia associated with haemodynamic compromise are at high risk of sudden death and should be treated with an automated implantable cardioverter defibrillator (ICD) as secondary prevention.

Information gained from the history, echocardiography, ambulatory electrocardiographic monitoring and exercise testing are used to risk stratify the remainder of patients.

Risk factors for sudden death in HCM are listed below. Unfortunately, the positive predictive value of these investigations is low, so confusion remains as to how patients with an abnormal test results should be treated. In general, individuals with two or more of the risk factors from Box 8.1 should be implanted with an ICD for primary prevention of a cardiac fatality. The negative predictive accuracy of these risk factors is excellent, therefore individuals without any recognized risk factors can be strongly reassured.

8.3 Arrhythmogenic right-ventricular cardiomyopathy

ARVC is a hereditary disease of heart muscle characterized by fibrofatty replacement of right-ventricular myocardium, ventricular arrhythmias and sudden death. It has been described in all ethnicities and both sexes. The prevalence of ARVC is between one per 1000 and one per 5000.

8.3.1 Aetiology

ARVC usually has autosomal dominant inheritance in 40–50%. Mutations in genes encoding several desmosomal proteins including plakoglobin, desmoplakin and desmoglein, are responsible for the disease process.

Box 8.1 Risk factors for premature sudden cardiac death in patients with HCM

- Unheralded syncope
- Family history of sudden death from HCM
- Severe (>30 mm) left-ventricular hypertrophy
- Severe left-ventricular obstruction (>60 mm Hg)
- Non-sustained ventricular tachycardia
- Abnormally flat blood pressure response to exercise

An autosomal recessive form of the disorder, Naxos disease that is characterized by plantarpalmar keratoderma and wooly hair appearance is also recognized.

8.3.2 Pathology

Macroscopically structural abnormalities in ARVC are initially subtle. The thinnest areas of the right-ventricular myocardium, notably the inflow and outflow tracts and the apex are first affected. As the disease progresses greater involvement of the right-ventricular free wall leads to right-ventricular aneurysms and dilatation of the cavity (see Figure 8.2). Left-ventricular involvement is becoming increasingly recognized.

The main histological feature is segmental transmural fibrofatty replacement of the normal myocardium. There maybe focal myocarditis and lymphocyte infiltration. Impaired cell adhesion leads to myocyte detachment and death. Following the initial inflammatory response myocytes are replaced with fibrofatty deposits which form the arrhythmogenic substrate that defines the disease.

8.3.3 Clinical features

Patients may present at any age with palpitations, presyncope or syncope, often precipitated by exercise. Symptoms usually represent ventricular arrhythmias. Rarely presentation can be as a result of right heart failure. Sudden cardiac death may be the first presentation particularly during exercise. Indeed ARVC is the commonest cause of sudden death during sport in Italy.

Classically the natural history of ARVC is considered to comprise of four distinct phases (see Table 8.2):

8.3.4 Investigating patients with suspected ARVC

Electrocardiography

The results of 12-lead electrocardiography are normal in up to 40% of patients with ARVC. T-wave inversion in the right-ventricular precordial leads (V1–V3) is characteristic. The QRS complex duration

Figure 8.2 Cross section of a heart showing gross right-ventricular dilation and transmural fibrofatty infiltration

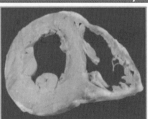

may be prolonged and show late potentials (epsilon waves) in V1–V3 suggestive of delayed right-ventricular depolarization (see Figure 8.3). Multiple ventricular ectopics of right-ventricular origin (left bundle branch block morphology) are common. The signal averaged electrocardiogram reveals late potentials in 50–80% of patients with ARVC.

Imaging

Echocardiography may be normal. In many circumstances, the abnormalities seen are subtle and detection is highly dependent upon operator experience. Intravenous contrast has been shown to enhance visualization of the right ventricle. Segmental wall motion abnormalities, aneurysm formation and gross dilatation of the right ventricle with generalized hypokinesia are features of advanced disease.

Magnetic resonance imaging is considered to be more sensitive for the identification of morphological right-ventricular changes associated with ARVC. However in the concealed phase of the disease the MRI may appear completely normal.

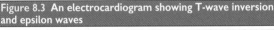

Table 8.2 Natural history of AVRC

Phase	Symptoms	Structural abnormalities
1. Concealed	Asymptomatic	None or mild
2. Overt arrhythmic	Symptomatic ventricular arrhythmias	Obvious right-ventricular wall involvement
3. Overt contractile	Right-ventricular failure	Gross dilatation of right ventricle
4. Advanced	Biventricular failure	Left-ventricular involvement

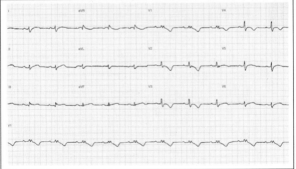

Figure 8.3 An electrocardiogram showing T-wave inversion and epsilon waves

Holter monitoring

Sustained or non-sustained ventricular tachycardia with a left bundle branch block morphology or frequent ventricular ectopy (>1000 ventricular ectopic beats in 24 hours) are well-recognized features of ARVC.

Exercise stress test

Increased frequency of ventricular ectopics or ventricular tachycardia during exercise may be helpful in the diagnosis of ARVC.

Right-ventricular biopsy

Histological diagnosis is rarely possible because the disease is patchy and a transmural biopsy is required.

Diagnosis

The diagnosis of ARVC is challenging for even the most able cardiologists and relies on a family history of ARVC and a plethora of electrocardiographic and cardiac imaging tests. Diagnostic criteria for index cases have been developed (see Table 8.3). The presence of two major, one major, and two minor or four minor criteria from different categories is considered diagnostic.

These criteria are highly specific but lack sensitivity meaning early disease often results in missed diagnoses. As relatives of a patient with ARVC have a 50% chance of carrying the mutated gene, less stringent criteria may be applied because abnormal results of investigations are more likely to represent disease expression.

8.3.5 **Treatment**

The aim of treatment is to relieve symptoms and to reduce the risk of sudden death. There is an association between sudden cardiac death and exercise and therefore competitive sports and training should be avoided.

ICDs are the most effective treatment of ventricular arrhythmias. They should be used in patients with ARVC who have survived a cardiac arrest or sustained ventricular arrhythmia for the purpose of secondary prevention. Beta-blockers and amiodarone should only be used as an adjunct to ICDs to suppress the frequency of ventricular arrhythmias. Heart failure should be treated using standard treatment.

8.3.6 **Risk stratification of patients with ARVC**

Several features have been shown to be associated with a high risk of sudden death and include young age at presentation, syncope, a family history of sudden cardiac death, right heart failure, left-ventricular involvement, QRS dispersion greater than 40 ms and certain mutations including Naxos disease. Patients with any of the above features should be considered for ICD implantation as primary prevention.

Table 8.3 International task force criteria for the diagnosis of AVRC

Major criteria	Minor criteria
Global and/or regional dysfunction and structural alteration • Severe dilatation and reduction of right-ventricular ejection fraction with no (or only mild) left-ventricular impairment • Localized right-ventricular aneurysms (akinetic or dyskinetic areas with diastolic bulging) • Severe segmental dilatation of the right ventricle	**Global and/or regional dysfunction and structural alteration** • Mild global right-ventricular dilatation and/or ejection fraction reduction with normal left ventricle • Mild segmental dilatation of the right ventricle • Regional right-ventricular hypokinesia
Tissue characterization of walls • Fibrofatty replacement of myocardium on endomyocardial biopsy	
	Repolarization abnormalities • Inverted T-waves in right precordial leads, V2 and V3 (people aged more than 12 ears; in the absence of right bundle branch block)
Depolarization conduction abnormalities • Epsilon waves or localized prolongation (>110ms) of the QRS complex in right precordial leads	**Depolarization or conduction abnormalities** • Late potentials on signal averaged ECG
	Arrhythmias • Left-bundle branch block-type ventricular tachycardia, sustained or non-sustained (electrocardiogram, Holter, exercise testing) • Frequent (>1000/24 hours) ventricular extra systole (Holter)
Family history • Family history confirmed at necropsy or surgery.	**Family history** • Family history of premature death (<35 years) due to suspected right-ventricular cardiomyopathy • Family history (clinical diagnosis based on these criteria

8.4 Familial dilated cardiomyopathy

Familial dilated cardiomyopathy is defined by dilatation and impaired left-ventricular systolic function in the absence of a known cause where two or more closely related relatives are affected. DCM has a prevalence of one per 2500 of which up to 35% is hereditary. Familial dilated cardiomyopathy has been described in patients of both sexes and all ethnic origins.

8.4.1 **Aetiology**

Inheritance is most commonly autosomal dominant though autosomal recessive, X-linked, and mitochondrial forms have been described. The proteins affected by mutations include: sarcomeric contractile proteins, cytoskeletal and sarcolemmal structural proteins, nuclear-envelope proteins, and proteins involved in cardiac energy metabolism.

DCM can be caused by mutations of genes encoding the same contractile proteins that are responsible for hypertrophic cardio-myopathy as well as proteins that form the sarcomeric structure including muscle LIM protein, α-actin-2, ZASP, and titin.

Mutations in the genes encoding the nuclear envelope proteins lamin A and lamin C are responsible for Emery-Dreifus muscular dystrophy. The muscular dystrophy is often slowly progressive and patients deteriorate because of heart failure from an associated DCM. This disease is also associated with heart block.

X-linked muscular dystrophies including Duchenne's (childhood) and Becker's (adult) are often associated with dilated cardiomyopathy. DCM associated with skeletal myopathy account for only 5% of cases.

Disorders that affect the fatty acid β-oxidation pathway and carnitine transport and metabolism can lead to dilated cardiomyopathy. These disorders usually have an autosomal recessive inheritance. Circumstances that increase the myocardial reliance upon fatty acids as an energy substrate e.g. fasting cause an accumulation of toxic metabolites that leads to myocardial damage.

Cardiomyopathy can occur in several disorders due to defects in mitochondrial oxidative phosphorylation. Neuromuscular disease is usually the prominent feature of these disorders. The disease-causing mutation is found on the mitochondrial genome.

8.4.2 **Pathology**

On macroscopic examination the enlarged heart often has increased mass, all four chambers may be dilated and there may be mural thrombi. Histological examination reveals myocyte hypertrophy and occasionally isolated inflammatory cells. These changes are non-specific and not suggestive of a particular cause.

8.4.3 **Clinical features**

Familial DCM can present at any age, though most commonly in the third and fourth decade of life. Initial presentation is often due to congestive cardiac failure. Family history and the presence of other phenotypic features, such as heart block (laminopathies), deafness or blindness (mitochondrial cytopathies), or neuromuscular weakness (neuron–cardiac syndromes), are useful in facilitating the correct diagnosis and further management.

Echocardiography confirms left-ventricular enlargement and systolic dysfunction. The treatment is identical to that of other causes of left-ventricular systolic dysfunction. As with other causes of dilated cardiomyopathy, the prognosis of familial cardiomyopathy is poor.

8.5 Hereditary infiltrative disorders causing cardiomyopathy

8.5.1 Familial cardiac amyloid

Mutations in the gene encoding transthyretin (TTR), a protein synthesized in the liver, are the commonest cause of familial amyloid disease. Over 100 mutations in the gene encoding TTR have been identified leading to abnormal folding of the protein and consequently the development of amyloidosis. Substitution of isoleucine for valine at position 122 (Val122Ile) is the commonest mutation and is found in 4% of African-Americans. Inheritance is autosomal dominant with a high degree of penetrance. The frequency of familial cardiac amyloid varies significantly with ethnicity. Its prevalence is believed to be 1.6% in African Americans compared with 0.4% in Caucasians.

8.5.2 Pathology

The amyloid protein subunits infiltrate the myocardium and form insoluble polymers or fibrils that adopt an antiparallel β-pleated sheet configuration. Deposits are found throughout the myocardium. The pericardium, cardiac valves, and coronary arteries may also be involved. As a result the myocardium becomes firm, rubbery, and non-compliant. There is thickening of the ventricular wall and cavities may become dilated.

8.5.3 Clinical features

The most common presentation is with symptoms of congestive cardiac failure.

Arrhythmias are common including atrial fibrillation and ventricular premature beats. Amyloid can infiltrate nodal and conducting tissue causing varying degrees of heart block. Isolated cardiac amyloid is rare and occurs in less than 5% if cases. As a consequence, extracardiac manifestations including neurological, renal, ocular, and cutaneous disease usually coexist.

8.5.4 Investigations

Electrocardiography

The electrocardiographic changes in cardiac amyloid are non-specific. Diminished voltages are seen in 50% of advanced cases and there may be loss of R waves in the precordial leads. Pseudoinfarct patterns (pathological q waves), heart block and atrial fibrillation are also recognized.

Imaging

Echocardiography shows increased thickness of the ventricular walls and reduced cavity size. The atria can be dilated. The myocardium has a characteristic 'speckled' appearance and the inter-atrial septum is bright. In early disease impaired relaxation and restrictive filling is the first abnormality seen. Systolic dysfunction occurs as disease progresses.

Late gadolinium enhancement on cardiac magnetic resonance imaging shows a characteristic pattern of global subendocardial enhancement.

Nuclear imaging can detect the distribution of radiolabelled serum amyloid protein. Imaging of hollow and moving organs is unreliable and therefore this investigation is not useful in detecting cardiac amyloid.

Biopsy

Endomyocardial biopsy is the gold-standard investigation in the diagnosis of cardiac amyloid. Sections of tissue stained with Congo red appear green in polarized light that is diagnostic of amyloid infiltration. Immunohistochemical staining can be performed which may help distinguish between different types of amyloidosis.

8.5.5 Treatment

Treatment of cardiac amyloid is usually supportive, though attempts to suppress expression of the abnormal amyloid protein can be made.

Symptomatic treatment of heart failure should be instituted. Caution is needed in the use of diuretic as they may exacerbate orthostatic hypotension in patients with autonomic dysfunction that may occur with neurological involvement. Digoxin and calcium antagonists selectively bind to amyloid fibrils and can have an enhanced effect. There is currently no specific treatment for familial cardiac amyloid.

8.5.6 Prognosis

Familial cardiac amyloidosis has a significantly better prognosis than cardiac involvement from AL and AA amyloidosis. Presentation is usually in the sixth or seventh decade and the mean survival is 72 months from time of diagnosis.

8.6 Fabry's disease

Fabry's disease is a rare systemic disorder caused by a deficiency in the enzyme α-galacosidase. It has X-linked inheritance and affects one in 40000 people. It is characterized by the intracellular accumulation of a glycolipid substrate in many organs including the heart, kidneys, skin, eyes, and the nervous system.

Cardiovascular manifestations include hypertension, mitral valve prolapse, heart failure, and arrhythmias. Physical examination often reveals angiokeratomas on the limbs and the perineal area. Slit-lamp examination of the eyes reveals characteristic changes in the cornea and retina.

Electrocardiography findings include abnormal p-wave morphology, conduction defects and left-ventricular hypertrophy. Echocardiography shows increase left-ventricular wall thickness. Cardiac magnetic resonance imaging and endomyocardial biopsy can help differentiate between other causes of hypertrophic and restrictive cardiomyopathies. Diagnosis is confirmed by the finding of low leucocyte α-galactosidase activity. Replacement of the enzyme shows mild improvement of left-ventricular function in some patients.

8.7 Left-ventricular non-compaction

LVNC is a disorder of endomyocardial morphogenesis characterized by marked trabeculations and intertrabecular recesses in the left-ventricular wall and depressed systolic function. It is a rare disorder with an unknown prevalence. The nomenclature of the disorder is misleading as the right ventricle is also commonly involved.

8.7.1 Aetiology

LVNC can be a hereditary. Several mutations encoding structural proteins including tafazzins, α-dystrobrevin, and Cypher/ZASP have been associated with the condition. The mode of inheritance has yet to be established. In children the disorder often coexists with other congenital abnormalities causing ventricular outflow obstruction such as aortic and pulmonary stenosis.

8.7.2 Pathology

Macroscopic examination reveals dilated ventricles with marked trabeculations and deep recesses (see Figure 8.4). During normal embryonic development, trabeculations occur at day 32 and invert by day 70. LVNC is believed to represent a failure in this compaction process resulting in non-compacted myocardium adjacent to the endocardium.

8.7.3 Clinical features

LVNC commonly presents with congestive cardiac failure. There is a high incidence of atrial and ventricular arrhythmias. Stagnation of blood in the intramural recesses predisposes to systemic emboli.

8.7.4 Investigations

Imaging techniques to identify trabeculations are the mainstay of investigation. Echocardiography, cardiac magnetic resonance imaging, cardiac computed tomography, and left ventriculogram have all been used to demonstrate a characteristic two layered appearance of the ventricular wall with perfusion into deep recesses. The inferior, lateral, and posterior walls are usually affected the most. Diagnosis is dependent upon the demonstration of hypertrabeculation, deep recesses and a ratio of non-compacted to compacted myocardium of two to one in end-systole.

8.7.5 Management

There is no specific treatment for LVNC. Therapy usually involves the treatment of heart failure. Anticoagulation is recommended to prevent systemic thromboembolism. Implantable cardioverter defibrillators are recommended in patients with poor systolic function and non-sustained or sustained ventricular tachycardia.

8.7.6 Prognosis

There have been claims based on small studies that the disorder has a worse prognosis than other cases of dilated cardiomyopathy; however, these claims are unfounded in subsequent evaluation of large cohorts. The natural history of the disorder is not yet well characterized.

8.8 Conclusion

Hereditary cardiomyopathies whilst rare should always be borne in mind when more conventional aetiologies do not account for the heart-failure syndrome. A range of different disorders requiring specialist input can present with different aspects of the heart failure syndrome. These often require sophisticated therapeutic approaches best managed by specialists in heart muscle disease.

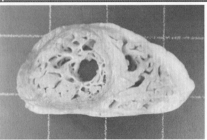

Figure 8.4 Heart showing marked trabeculations in the left- and right-ventricular wall characteristic of left-ventricular non-compaction

Key references

Maron, B., Towbin, J., Thiene, G., *et al.* (2006). Contemporary definitions and classification of the cardiomyopathies. *Circulation*, **113**, 1807–16.

Elliott, P., McKenna, W. (2004). Hypertrophic cardiomyopathy. *Lancet*, **9424**, 1881–91.

Elliott, P (2007). Investigation and treatment of hypertrophic cardiomyopathy. *Clin. Med.*, **7**, 383–7.

Spirito, P., Seidman, C., McKenna, W., Maron, B. (1997). The management of hypertrophic cardiomyopathy. *N. Engl. J. Med.*, **336**, 775–85.

Sen-Chowdhry, S., Lowe, M., Sporton, S., McKenna, W. (2004). Arrhythmogenic right-ventricular cardiomyopathy: clinical presentation, diagnosis and management. *Am. J. Med.*, **117**, 685–95.

Gemayel, C., Pelliccia, A., Thompson, P. (2001). Arrhythmogenic right-ventricular cardiomyopathy. *J. Am. Coll. Cardiol.*, **38**, 1773–81.

Burkitt, E., Hershberger, R. (2005). Clinical and genetic issues in familial dilated cardiomyopathy. *J. Am. Coll. Cardiol.*, **45**, 969–81.

Falk, R. (2005). Diagnosis and management of cardiac amyloidoses. *Circulation*, **112**, 2047–60.

Jenni, R., Oechslin, E., Van der Loo, B. (2007). Isolated ventricular non-compaction of the myocardium in adults. *Heart*, **93**, 11–5.

Chapter 9

Chronic heart failure with preserved ejection fraction

Gilles W. De Keulenaer and Dirk L. Brutsaert

> **Key Points**
> - Chronic heart failure with preserved ejection fraction is as common as chronic heart failure with reduced ejection fraction.
> - After hospitalization for heart failure with preserved ejection fraction, prognosis and rehospitalization rates are comparable to heart failure with reduced ejection fraction.
> - Systolic function of the cardiac muscle is impaired in heart failure with preserved ejection fraction.
> - According to a recent consensus statement of the Heart Failure Association of the European Society of Cardiology, the diagnosis of heart failure with preserved ejection fraction remains challenging, but the use of serum brain natriuretic peptide (BNP) and tissue Doppler imaging (TDI) has increased accuracy.
> - Treatment of heart failure with preserved ejection fraction should be empiric, and phenotype-oriented as well as symptom-oriented.

9.1 Epidemiological background

As discussed in Chapter 2, heart failure is a clinical syndrome characterized by symptoms and signs of decreased tissue perfusion and increased tissue water. Although often associated with severe left-ventricular-pump dysfunction and a reduced left-ventricular ejection fraction (LVEF), this syndrome can occur at any LVEF. In fact, recent surveys have shown a unimodal distribution of LVEF ranging from 10% to 90%, when measured in a large group of patients hospitalized for heart failure (see Figure 9.1).

Despite the unimodal distribution of LVEF, heart failure has been dogmatically subdivided in two groups depending on whether ejection fraction is lower than 50%, so called "systolic heart failure", or equal to or higher than 50%, so called "diastolic heart failure" or "heart failure with a normal ejection fraction" (HFNEF). The number of patients hospitalized with HFNEF has been steadily increasing over the past 20 years, whereas the number of admissions for heart failure with reduced ejection fraction has not changed (see Figure 9.2).

The reasons for these shifting epidemiological data of chronic heart failure are multifaceted. The data may reveal a genuine increase in HFNEF, reflecting the current ageing of western populations as well as the increasing prevalence of atrial fibrillation, obesity, diabetes, and hypertension, factors that are commonly associated with HFNEF. Increased survival after acute coronary syndromes and introduction

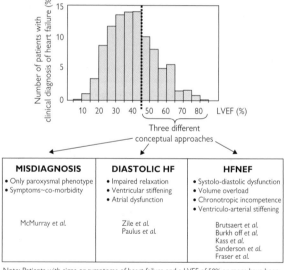

Figure 9.1 **Unimodal distribution of LVEF in chronic heart failure revealed in the heart failure surveys I and II of the European Society of Cardiology**

Three different conceptual approaches

MISDIAGNOSIS	DIASTOLIC HF	HFNEF
• Only paroxysmal phenotype • Symptoms~co-morbidity	• Impaired relaxation • Ventricular stiffening • Atrial dysfunction	• Systolo-diastolic dysfunction • Volume overload • Chronotropic incompetence • Ventriculo-arterial stiffening
McMurray et al.	Zile et al. Paulus et al.	Brutsaert et al. Burkh off et al. Kass et al. Sanderson et al. Fraser et al.

Note: Patients with signs or symptoms of heart failure and a LVEF of 50% or more have been dogmatically differentiated from other patients with heart failure and systematically excluded from clinical trials. Controversy remains on the severity, natural history, and pathophysiology of the disease with different conceptual approaches by at least three scientific movements.

of efficient oral medication, such as angiotensin-converting-enzyme inhibitors and beta-blockers, given as preventive therapies against LV remodelling to patients with hypertension or coronary artery disease, may also have contributed. The observed increase in HFNEF may, in addition, reflect a growing awareness by the physician. Whereas previously the diagnosis of heart failure was challenged when LVEF fraction was preserved, the evolving concept of diastolic dysfunction and the simultaneous introduction of blood-flow Doppler, tissue Doppler echocardiography, and serum brain natriuretic peptide (BNP) assays have increased the propensity to diagnose heart failure regardless of LVEF.

9.2 Remaining controversies about HFNEF

HFNEF is subject to ongoing discussions and many conceptual controversies remain (see Figure 9.1). Some clinicians claim that HFNEF is manifested only as a paroxysmal disease, e.g. during episodes of hypertensive crises or episodes of atrial fibrillation, but that chronic symptoms such as shortness of breath, ankle edema and paroxysmal nocturnal dyspnea usually require another explanation (related to obesity and respiratory disease). They argue that many patients are erroneously diagnosed as suffering from HFNEF based on an isolated finding of diastolic dysfunction on Doppler echocardiography.

Other investigators, however, agree that HFNEF is a common explanation for chronic heart failure but they disagree about the underlying pathophysiology (see Table 9.1). A first school defends the theory that HFNEF is completely explained by diastolic LV dysfunction occurring as an isolated manifestation. This school has coined the

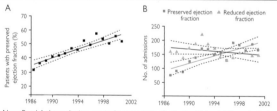

Figure 9.2 Increasing prevalence or increasing awareness of heart failure with preserved ejection fraction

Note: Panel A shows the increase in the percentage of patients with heart failure who had preserved ejection fraction. Panel B shows that the number of admissions for heart failure with preserved ejection fraction increased during the past 15 years, whereas the number of admissions for heart failure with reduced ejection fraction did not change.

Figure 9.2 is reproduced with permission from Owan TE, Hodge DO, Herges RM, *et al.* 2006. Trends in prevalence and outcome of heart failure with preserved ejection fraction. *N. Engl. J. Med.*, **355**: 251–9.

term "diastolic heart failure" in an attempt to underline the, in their opinion, unique physiological characteristics of the disease—i.e. diastolic dysfunction either caused by intrinsic impairment of LV relaxation usually combined with ventricular stiffening or secondary to ventricular stiffening or to atrial dysfunction. To them, HFNEF would then be a syndrome to be distinguished from "systolic heart failure."

A second scientific mainstream interprets HFNEF in a much broader pathophysiological context, mainly defending the view that HFNEF is not essentially different from systolic heart failure. From this pathophysiological point of view HFNEF is then considered rather as a "variant clinical phenotype" of heart failure in which combined systolo-diastolic dysfunctions (including LV relaxation impairment and ventriculoarterial stiffening), volume overload and sympathovagal imbalances play a role. The recent observation that the Kaplan-Meier survival curves of HFNEF and systolic heart failure completely overlap is consistent with this conjecture. HFNEF is then used as a mere descriptive term, useful in a clinical context, but pathophysiologically insignificant. For clarity of the reader, this chapter will be continued in the spirit of the latter view.

Table 9.1 Heart failure: a single or two syndromes?	
Heart failure evolves as a *single syndrome* with HF with normal LVEF preceding HF with reduced LVEF	Heart failure evolves as *two syndromes*, one with concentric LV remodelling and mainly diastolic LV dysfunction (DHF) and one with eccentric LV remodelling and combined systolo-diastolic dysfunction (SHF)
Arguments	*Arguments*
1. Unimodal distribution of LVEF in HF trials 2. Continuous decline of TD LV long axis shortening velocity from HFNEF to HFREF 3. Progression to eccentric LV remodelling in hypertensive heart disease especially in African and Asian populations 4. Progression to eccentric LV remodelling in endstage hypertrophic cardiomyopathy	1. Presence of concentric LV remodelling in DHF and eccentric LV remodelling in SHF 2. Distinct myocardial ultrastructure with prominent cardiomyocyte hypertrophy in DHF and reduced myofilamentary density in SHF 3. Higher in-vitro cardiomyocyte resting tension in DHF 4. Distinct isoform shifts of the cytoskeletal protein titin 5. Distinct expression pattern of matrix metalloproteinases and tissue inhibitors of matrix metalloproteinases 6. Prognostic improvement under current heart failure therapy in SHF but not in DHF

Table 9.1 is reproduced with permission from Paulus, WJ, Tschope, C, Sanderson, JE, *et al.* (2007). How to diagnose diastolic heart failure. *Eur. Heart J.*, **28**: 2539–50.

9.3 **Pathophysiology of heart failure with preserved ejection fraction**

HFNEF can be defined as a clinical syndrome characterized by symptoms and signs of heart failure, a preserved ejection fraction and diastolic failure. Importantly, from our perspective, a preserved ejection fraction indicates that the systolic performance of the ventricle, as a haemodynamic pump, is preserved. The systolic function of the ventricle as a muscular pump may, however, already be compromised significantly, as demonstrated by numerous, mainly echo-Doppler based studies and the application of tissue Doppler technology. It is therefore inaccurate to state that HFNEF is a syndrome with preserved systolic ventricular function.

Diastolic failure occurs when the ventricular chamber is unable to accept an adequate volume of blood during diastole at normal diastolic pressures and volumes sufficient to maintain an appropriate stroke volume. These abnormalities are caused by impaired systolic ventricular relaxation (induced either by an excessive external load or by abnormal inactivation processes, or by abnormal paracrine endothelial or endocrine signalling) or decreased ventricular compliance (induced by cytoskeletal or extracellular matrix abnormalities or by abnormal paracrine endothelial signalling). In addition, there is emerging evidence that volume overload, as well as ventriculoarterial stiffening, may play a role. Although these disturbances may result in higher filling pressures at rest; they more frequently produce elevated filling pressures during exercise, which results in exercise dyspnoea.

It may be important to remember that LV relaxation abnormalities, as commonly observed in HFNEF, should be interpreted from within an appropriate conceptual-physiological approach to cardiac performance. As elaborated in more detail in Figure 9.3, the heart can be perceived either as a hydraulic–hemodynamic pump or as a muscular pump. From the perspective of the heart as a muscular pump—in which essential functional muscular aspects of the heart, such as time of onset of LV relaxation, ventricular twisting and untwisting, differences between long-axis and radial-axis fibre shorting, and myocardial strain and strain rate are taken into account—isovolumic relaxation and even early rapid filling are an intrinsic part of the contraction–relaxation cycle of cardiac muscle "systole", with impaired relaxation being the manifestation of dysfunction of cardiac-muscle systole. The strong linear correlations between impaired myocardial velocities during contraction and relaxation in a large group of patients with and without heart failure are consistent with this view.

Figure 9.3 Heart failure with preserved ejection fraction is a manifestation of systolo-diastolic dysfunction of the LV muscle-pump

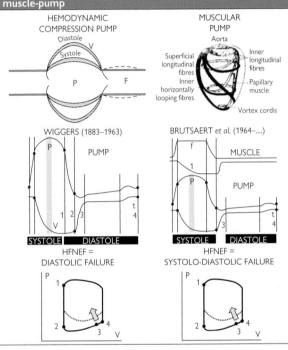

9.4 Clinical manifestations of heart failure with preserved ejection fraction

The classic findings of systolic heart failure are pulmonary congestion and high venous pressure; these are equally manifestations of HFNEF. Hence, differentiation between systolic and diastolic heart failure cannot be made on the basis of history, physical examination, electro-cardiogram, or chest X-ray alone because markers of these examinations occur with the same relative frequency in both disease states.

As mentioned above, however, epidemiological studies have revealed that HFNEF generally occurs at an older age (HFNEF is rare below the age of 50 years), and more frequently affects women and obese people (see Table 9.2). Conditions associated with and likely contributing to the development of HFNEF include hypertension, LV hypertrophy, and diabetes mellitus.

In a recent prospective multicentre registry in the New York metropolitan area on 619 patients hospitalized for decompensated HFNEF, it was observed that the precipitating factors for hospitalizations consisted of hypertension (13%), non-compliance to therapy (12.8%), renal insufficiency (9%), and atrial fibrillation (9%). Two or more precipitating factors were present in 19.3% of patients. Importantly, 85% of patients had chronic overt symptoms of heart failure that antedated hospitalization. Also, re-hospitalization frequency of HFNEF was high, with rates being similar for HFNEF and systolic heart failure (6 month all-cause readmission rate 45%).

Table 9.2 Characteristics of patients with heart failure with preserved or reduced ejection fraction

Characteristic	Reduced Ejection Fraction (N = 2429)	Preserved Ejection Fraction (N = 2167)	P Value	Adjusted P Value
Age (yr)	71.7±12.1	74.4±14.4	<0.001	NA
Male sex (% of patients)	65.4	44.3	<0.001	<0.001
Body-mass index	28.6±7.0	29.7±7.8	0.002	0.17
Obesity (% of patients)	35.5	41.4	0.007	0.002
Serum creatinine on admission (mg/dl)	1.6±1.0	1.6±1.1	0.31	0.30
Hemoglobin on admission (g/dl)	12.5±2.0	11.8±2.1	<0.001	<0.001
Hypertension (% of patients)	48.0	62.7	<0.001	<0.001
Coronary artery disease (% of patients)	63.7	52.9	<0.001	<0.001
Atrial fibrillation (% of patients)	28.5	41.3	<0.001	<0.001
Diabetes (% of patients)	34.3	33.1	0.42	0.61
Substantial valve disease (% of patients)	6.5	2.6	<0.001	0.05
Ejection fraction (%)	29±10	61±7	<0.001	NA

Table 9.2 is reproduced with permission from Owan TE, Hodge DO, Herges RM, et al. 2006. Trends in prevalence and outcome of heart failure with preserved ejection fraction. N. Engl. J. Med., **355**: 251–9.

Patients with HFNEF have a worse prognosis than age-matched controls without heart failure. In fact, several recent surveys have established that the post-discharge risk for mortality is not different from patients with systolic heart failure (up to 10% mortality at 3 months, 30% at 1 year, and 65% at 5 years; see Figure 9.4). Importantly, however, little information is available on the cause of death of patients with HFNEF. Given the important number of coexisting illnesses of these patients, these data are urgently needed to predict better the nature and benefit of treatment. Interestingly, in a subgroup of 375 patients with mean LVEF of 64% who were participating in the PEP-CHF trial (Perindopril in Elderly People with Chronic Heart Failure), serum levels of NT-pro-BNP identified patients at high risk for death or hospitalization related to heart failure (see Figure 9.4).

9.5 **Diagnosis of heart failure with preserved ejection fraction**

Although impaired systolic relaxation and genuine diastolic abnormalities may undoubtedly contribute to symptoms of heart failure in patients with HFNEF, their relative contribution to the symptoms in an individual patient remains challenging. For example, slow LV relaxation is observed on transmitral Doppler echocardiography in about 70% of individuals over the age of 75 years, but only a small fraction has clinical signs of heart failure. There is a clear need for clinically useful criteria for attributing suspect heart failure clinical symptoms to LV diastolic dysfunction in the presence of a preserved LVEF.

As for diagnostic criteria for HFNEF, the Heart Failure Association of the European Society of Cardiology proposed that three obligatory conditions should be satisfied simultaneously (the Paulus criteria):

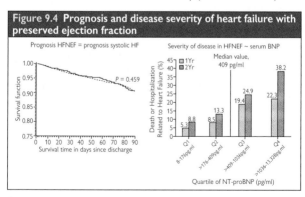

Figure 9.4 Prognosis and disease severity of heart failure with preserved ejection fraction

Figure 9.4 is reproduced with permission from Fonarow *et al.* (2007). *J. Am. Coll. Cardiol.*, **50**: 768–77 (left panel) and from Cleland *et al.* (2007). *N. Engl. J. Med.*, **357**: 829–30 (right panel).

1) presence of signs or symptoms of congestive heart failure; 2) presence of normal or mildly abnormal LV systolic function; 3) evidence of abnormal ventricular relaxation, filling, diastolic distensibility, or diastolic stiffness. These criteria are based on a previous statement paper by the European Society of Cardiology, which has now been revised. As specified in Figure 9.5, the third criterion can be obtained invasively, with tissue Doppler, or by showing elevated levels of natriuretic peptides combined with blood flow Doppler, tissue Doppler or some 2D echo evidence of LV hypertrophy or atrial dilatation. These criteria certainly help in daily cardiology and in the design of future clinical trials on HFNEF, but still need to be validated with regard to their diagnostic accuracy. In line with the above pathophysiological considerations, the three criteria should, in our opinion, be slightly reformulated. In Figure 9.6, a flow chart, as formulated by the European Heart Failure Association, on how to exclude HFNEF is also shown.

9.6 Treatment of heart failure with preserved ejection fraction

Randomized multicentre trials in patients with HFNEF are scarce and only a few are still ongoing. The recommendations for the management of HFNEF are, therefore, based on small clinical studies lacking a pathophysiological concept and validated diagnostic guidelines. Treatment of HFNEF should essentially be directed at two goals: reducing symptoms and improving prognosis by targeting the mechanisms of disease.

9.6.1 Symptom-targeted treatment

Diastolic pressure can be reduced by decreasing ventricular volume with diuretics, venodilators, or neurohormonal inhibitors, by restoring heart rate to normal, by reducing blood pressure, and by maintaining synchronous atrial contraction. Doses of diuretics should be relatively low when initiated since a small change in diastolic volume may cause a large change in pressure and cardiac output and may lead to hypotension. An additional advantage of modulating the neurohormonal system may be that it also affects fibroblast activity and fibrosis, calcium handling and myocardial stiffness.

Reducing heart rate in HFNEF may have a double-edged effect. On the one hand, it may have a beneficial impact on ischaemia-related diastolic dysfunction and may avoid the problem of incomplete relaxation seen at high heart rates. On the other hand, blunting exercise-induced increases in heart rates may also inappropriately inhibit an important mechanism of the (hypertrophic) heart to increase

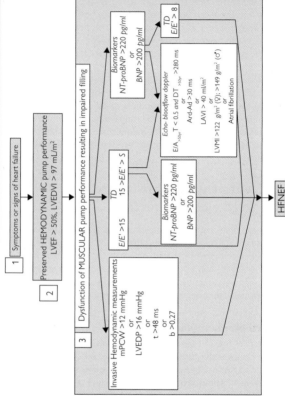

Figure 9.5 Modified flow chart for diagnosis of HFNEF according to the Heart Failure Association of the European Society of Cardiology

Note: LVEDVI = left-ventricular end-diastolic volume index; mPCW = mean pulmonary capillary wedge pressure; LVEDP = left-ventricular end-diastolic pressure; τ = time constant of left-ventricular relaxation; b = constant of left-ventricular chamber stiffness; TD = tissue Doppler; E = early mitral-valve flow velocity; E' = early TD lengthening velocity; NT-proBNP = n terminal-pro brain natriuretic peptide; BNP = brain natriuretic peptide; E/A = ratio of early (E) to late (A) mitral-valve flow velocity; DT = deceleration time; LVMI = left-ventricular mass index; LAVI = left atrial volume index; Ard = duration of reverse pulmonary vein atrial systole flow; Ad = duration of mitral valve atrial wave flow.

Figure 9.5 reproduced in modified form from Paulus, WJ, Tschope, C, Sanderson, JE, et al. (2007). How to diagnose diastolic heart failure. *Eur. Heart. J.*, **28**: 2539–50.

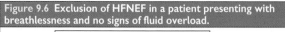

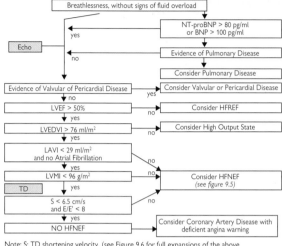

Figure 9.6 Exclusion of HFNEF in a patient presenting with breathlessness and no signs of fluid overload.

Note: S: TD shortening velocity. (see Figure 9.6 for full expansions of the above abbreviations).

cardiac output, especially since some of these hearts manifest a small recruitable inotropic and preload reserve and thus rely on chronotropy for adaptations of cardiac output to peripheral demands

9.6.2 Mechanism-targeted treatment

Randomized clinical trials on mechanism-targeted treatment in HFNEF have been slow to develop. The main reasons for this delay have been a lack of recognition of the importance of HFNEF, a lack of consensus on the underlying pathophysiology, a lack of appropriate diagnostic criteria, and a perception that the investment for funding of studies is not commercially interesting. None of the trials specifically targeting HFNEF has, thus far, shown a significant effect of either digoxin, angiotensin-converting-enzyme inhibitors, or angiotensin-receptor inhibitors on overall mortality (see Table 9.3).

In the DIG EF (heart failure with LVEF greater than 45% and sinus rhythm required) digoxin induced a significant reduction in heart failure hospitalizations, but a trend towards more hospitalizations for non-heart failure hospitalizations. In the CHARM-preserved trial

Figure 9.6 is reproduced with permission from Paulus WJ, Tschope C, Sanderson JE, et al. 2007. How to diagnose diastolic heart failure. *Eur. Heart. J.*, **28**: 2539–50.

Table 9.3 Clinical trials of heart failure with preserved ejection fraction

Trial name	Intervention	Key entry criteria	Effect on mortality	Effect on HF-related hospitalizations
DIG (NEjM 1997)	Digoxin	• EF >40% • NYHA II–IV • sinus rhythm	No significant effect	Significant reduction
CHARM-preserved (The Lancet 2003)	Candesartan	• EF >40% • NYHA II–IV	No significant effect	Significant reduction
I-PRESERVE	Irbesartan	• EF >45% • age >60 • NYHA II–IV	To be reported	To be reported
PEP-CHF (Eur Heart J 2006)	Perindopril	• Age >70 • clinical and echo criteria of HF • mean EF = 65%	No significant effect	Significant reduction
SENIORS (Eur Heart J 2005)	Nebivolol	• Age >70 • EF <35% or HF hospitalization within 6 months	No significant effect	Not reported

(heart failure with LVEF higher than 40%, but patient characteristics strongly diverging from HFNEF patients in the community) candesartan had a moderate but significant impact by preventing hospital admissions for heart failure. Similarly, in the PEP-CHF trial, a trial in elderly people with rather milder degrees of HFNEF (mean LVEF 65%), perindopril did not reduce overall mortality, perhaps because of low event rates (4% per year), but significantly reduced hospitalizations for heart failure.

In some recent heart-failure trials, inclusion criteria no longer include limitations for LVEF, thereby studying heart failure over the whole spectrum of LVEF. In one such trials, the SENIORS trial, nebivolol reduced the composite endpoint of death or cardiovascular hospitalization, but the modest trend towards improved mortality did not reach statistical significance.

9.7 Conclusions

HFNEF is a common disorder and frequent cause of hospital admission, readmission, and mortality. Whilst there are many data and a multitude of randomized controlled trials for patients with CHF and reduced ejection fraction, such depth of data and understanding is lacking in HFNEF. At present treatment is based on pathophysiology rather than therapeutic long-term studies. Such studies are becoming more important as ageing, obesity, and diabetes are important correlates of HFNEF.

Key references

Owan, T.E., Hodge, D.O., Herges, R.M., Jacobsen, S.J., Roger, V.L., Redfield, M.M. (2006). Trends in prevalence and outcome of heart failure with preserved ejection fraction. *N. Engl. J. Med.*, **355**, 251–9.

De Keulenaer, G.W., Brutsaert, D.L. (2007). Systolic and diastolic heart failure: different phenotypes of the same disease? *Eur. J. Heart Fail.*, **9**, 136–43.

Sanderson, J.E. (2007). Heart failure with a normal ejection fraction. *Heart*, **93**, 155–8.

Maurer, M.S., Kronzon, I., Burkhoff, D. (2006). Ventricular pump function in heart failure with normal ejection fraction: insights from pressure-volume measurements. *Prog. Cardiovasc. Dis.*, **49**, 182–95.

Brutsaert, D.L. (2006). Cardiac dysfunction in heart failure: the cardiologist's love affair with time. *Prog. Cardiovasc. Dis.*, **49**,157–81.

Paulus, W.J., Tschope, C., Sanderson, J.E., *et al.* (2007). How to diagnose diastolic heart failure: a consensus statement on the diagnosis of heart failure with normal left-ventricular ejection fraction by the Heart Failure and Echocardiography Associations of the European Society of Cardiology. *Eur. Heart. J.*, **28**, 2539–50.

Chapter 10

Comorbidities associated with chronic heart failure

Alan Japp and David Newby

Key Points
• In patients with chronic heart failure (CHF), non-cardiac comorbidities exacerbate symptoms, worsen prognosis, and complicate treatment.
• Targeting associated comorbid conditions in CHF may offer novel avenues for treatment.
• In the absence of a genuine contraindication, patients with CHF and chronic obstructive pulmonary disease should be prescribed beta-blocker therapy.
• Continuous-positive-airway-pressure therapy relieves symptoms in patients with CHF and sleep-disordered breathing but does not improve CHF-related clinical outcomes.
• Recombinant erythropoietin represents a promising treatment for CHF patients with anaemia and merits further assessment in large-scale randomized controlled trials.

99

10.1 Background

Chronic heart failure (CHF) is frequently complicated by a number of chronic non-cardiac conditions (see Box 10.1). These tend to be particularly prevalent in the elderly who comprise the majority of patients with CHF (see Chapter 11). In addition to the obvious impact on symptoms and quality of life, the presence of comorbidities in patients with CHF carries important implications for prognosis and treatment. The total number of associated comorbidities correlates strongly with the risk of hospitalization, and many comorbidities independently predict the risk of death.

Comorbidities may complicate the treatment of CHF, particularly in frail, elderly patients. Such patients are often excluded from major clinical trials, and treatment has to be extrapolated from younger and unrepresentative populations. Moreover adherence to standard therapeutic regimens leads inevitably to polypharmacy and the potential for multiple drug interactions. Nevertheless, the identification and treatment of these disorders can have a favourable impact on symptoms, quality of life and prognosis. Furthermore there is emerging evidence that targeting specific comorbidities may influence the progression of heart failure, thereby opening up new avenues for treatment.

Box 10.1 Common non-cardiac comorbidities in CHF

- Anaemia
- Asthma
- COPD and bronchiectasis
- Renal dysfunction

- Arthritis
- Cognitive dysfunction
- Depression

10.2 **Chronic obstructive pulmonary disease**

Between one-quarter and one-third of patients with CHF meet diagnostic criteria for chronic obstructive pulmonary disease (COPD). This association is largely driven by the common aetiological factors of ageing and smoking. In addition patients with advanced COPD may develop pulmonary hypertension leading to the development of right-ventricular hypertrophy and failure (cor pulmonale).

Patients with CHF exhibit a restrictive ventilatory defect and impaired lung diffusion, while COPD is characterized by progressive airflow obstruction and destruction of lung tissue. The combination of these disorders may therefore result in severely impaired lung function and patients frequently have severe dyspnoea and exercise limitation. The presence of COPD in patients with CHF is associated with greater cardiovascular morbidity including non-fatal myocardial infarction, stroke, and hospitalization as well as higher mortality rates.

The coexistence of CHF and COPD presents diagnostic difficulties. In both conditions, the predominant symptom is exertional breathlessness with exercise limitation and there is often overlap of other clinical features, especially with cor pulmonale. The identification of CHF in patients with COPD poses particular challenges. Hyperinflation of the lungs may obscure characteristic physical signs (e.g. third heart sound), diminish chest X-ray findings (e.g. cardiomegaly), and limit echocardiographic assessment. Elevated serum brain natriuretic peptide (BNP) concentrations are usually helpful in distinguishing CHF from other causes of dyspnoea but are also increased in cor pulmonale. MRI may provide a more accurate means of assessing cardiac performance than echocardiography in patients with hyperinflation of the chest (see Chapter 3).

COPD frequently results in suboptimal heart-failure therapy. Beta-blockers are among the most effective treatments in CHF (see Chapter 6), but are commonly withheld in patients with concomitant COPD for fear of precipitating or aggravating bronchospasm. However, extensive evidence including a recent meta-analysis suggests cardioselective beta-blockers are safe in COPD and do not exacerbate respiratory symptoms, reduce forced expiratory volume in the first second (FEV_1) or impair response to inhaled bronchodilators, even in patients with significant reversibility or severe airflow limitation. In the absence of a genuine contraindication, patients with CHF and COPD should be prescribed beta-blocker therapy.

10.3 Sleep disordered breathing

The presence of sleep-disordered breathing is at least twice as common in patients with CHF than the general population and may take the form of either central or obstructive sleep apnoea.

10.3.1 Obstructive sleep apnoea/hypopnoea syndrome

Obstructive sleep apnoea/hypopnoea syndrome (OSAHS) is caused by recurrent complete or partial occlusion of the pharynx during sleep. Patients feel unrefreshed after sleep and experience daytime somnolence, often accompanied by impaired concentration and irritability. These symptoms may compound the CHF symptoms of fatigue, tiredness, and listlessness associated with a low cardiac output and have an

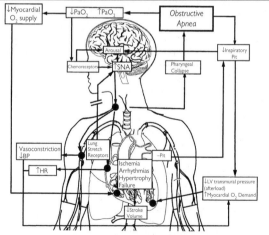

Figure 10.1 The pathophysiological consequences of apnoeic episodes in OSAHS on the cardiovascular system

Note: 1) The effort of trying to breathe against an occluded pharynx generates high negative intrathoracic pressures, greatly increasing loading of the ventricles. 2) Intermittent hypoxaemia may impair cardiac contractility, increase pulmonary arterial pressure and exacerbate myocardial ischaemia. 3) Recurrent cycle of apnoeas and arousals results in excessive sympathetic nervous system activation and consequent surges of blood pressure. OSAHS = obstructive sleep apnoea/hypopnoea syndrome. 4) Pit = intrathoracic pressure.

Figure 10.1 is reproduced from Bradley TD, *et al.* 2003. *Circulation*, **107**: 1671–8, with permission from the American Heart Association.

adverse impact on cardiovascular physiology (see Figure 10.1). Pathophysiological consequences of OSAHS include hypertension, increased oxidative stress, impaired endothelial function and left-ventricular hypertrophy. Patients with CHF and OSAHS have a two-fold greater mortality risk that those with CHF alone.

Continuous positive airways pressure (CPAP) is effective in relieving symptoms of OSAHS and produces physiological benefits including reduced nocturnal hypoxaemia and improved control of hypertension. In patients with both OSAHS and CHF, CPAP improves symptoms, but it remains unclear whether CPAP enhances cardiac performance in this setting. In the absence of definitive evidence we would not recommend CPAP therapy in CHF patients with asymptomatic OSAHS.

10.3.2 **Central sleep apnoea**

Central sleep apnoea (CSA) results from either a reduction in central respiratory drive or instability in feedback control of the central respiratory centre. The latter is common in patients with CHF who are predisposed to hyperventilation through stimulation of lung vagal irritant receptors during pulmonary congestion and exaggerated ventilatory responsiveness to carbon dioxide (see Figure 10.2). The prevalence of CSA has declined with the advent of modern CHF treatments; whilst early prevalence studies suggested it was as high as 40%, contemporary studies suggest a figure of less than 5%. Recurrent apnoeas lead to nocturnal hypoxaemia and intermittent sympathetic surges but without the negative intrathoracic pressures and consequent adverse loading conditions associated with OSAHS. CSA is associated with an increased risk of arrhythmias in patients with CHF, but it is not yet clear whether it contributes to mortality independently of other risk factors. No treatments specifically targeting CSA in CHF patients have yet been shown to improve clinical outcomes. A recent randomized trial of CPAP in 258 patients with CHF and CSA showed modest improvement in several physiological variables but failed to demonstrate major benefit on morbidity or mortality.

10.4 **Chronic kidney disease**

Around 40% of patients with CHF have an estimated glomerular filtration rate (GFR) of less than 60 ml per min per 1.73 m^2. The high prevalence of chronic kidney disease (CKD) in CHF patients results mainly from renal hypoperfusion and important common risk factors including hypertension and diabetes mellitus. Primary renal disease is also associated with accelerated atherosclerosis, fluid retention, and hypertension and this may precipitate or worsen myocardial dysfunction. In patients in whom the two disorders coexist, it can be difficult to determine the relative contributions to fluid overload from intrinsic kidney disease and impaired left-ventricular function.

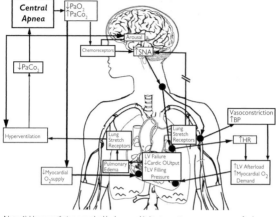

Figure 10.2 Pathophysiological mechanisms by which CHF leads to CSA

Note: 1) Hyperventilation provoked by lung vagal irritant receptors as consequence of pulmonary congestion. 2) $PaCO_2$ falls below apnoeic threshold leading to transient cessation of breathing 3) Upon subsequent rise in $PaCO_2$, oversensitivity of chemoreceptors leads to exaggerated ventilatory response and 'overshoot' of $PaCO_2$ below apnoeic threshold establishing vicious circle.

103

The presence of CKD in patients with CHF is an independent predictor of poor outcomes including death and hospitalization with heart failure. The prognostic value of renal dysfunction is of a similar magnitude to NYHA class and left-ventricular ejection fraction, and extends to patients with heart failure who have preserved left-ventricular systolic function. Several mechanisms have been postulated to account for this association. The increased risk is not fully explained by either the greater haemodynamic impairment seen in patients with advanced heart failure or the accelerated atherosclerosis that occurs in renal failure. Another leading explanation is that the anaemia resulting from reduced production of erythropoietin in CKD may accelerate the progression of heart failure.

The coexistence of CKD with CHF presents diagnostic and therapeutic challenges. Serum BNP concentrations tend to be increased independently in CKD; consequently a higher BNP threshold of 200 pg per ml should be used when estimated GFR is less than 60 ml per min per $1.73m^2$. There is also an overlap in physical signs with fluid overload and pulmonary oedema seen in both conditions. Patients can be resistant to diuretics and higher doses may be required to avoid fluid overload. The risk of digitalis toxicity is increased, and patients taking digoxin should have serum concentrations monitored and adjusted. The mortality and morbidity benefits of angiotensin-converting-enzyme inhibitors and angiotensin-receptor blockers in CHF extend to patients with renal impairment and these agents may also confer direct renoprotective effects. However, their use in patients with CKD carries a greater risk of acute deterioration in renal function in the context of hypovolaemia as well as serious electrolyte disturbance. In general an attempt should be made to use these agents though cautiously. Where their use is not possible, combined treatment with hydralazine and nitrate offers an alternative evidence-based strategy. The use of spironolactone is not recommended in patients with a serum creatinine greater than 220 mmol per litre or potassium greater than 5 mmol per litre due to the increased risk of serious renal dysfunction and hyperkalaemia. However, in patients with moderate-to-severe CHF who have mild renal impairment spironolactone may be used in low doses (25–50 mg) provided renal function and electrolytes are monitored closely and the drug is promptly discontinued in the event of rising concentrations of creatinine or potassium. Finally, there is strong evidence that the use of beta-blockers reduces mortality and morbidity even in patients with moderate to severe renal impairment and those with end-stage renal disease receiving haemodialysis.

10.5 **Chronic anaemia**

Anaemia is a very common comorbid condition in patients with CHF. Using the World Health Organization definition of anaemia as a plasma haemoglobin concentration less than 12 g per dl in women and less than 13 g per dl in men, the prevalence of anaemia in CHF ranges from 20% to 55%. Several different mechanisms underpin this association and the aetiology is often multfactorial (see Figure 10.3).

In patients with CHF, anaemia is associated with a poorer quality of life, more severe symptoms (especially exercise intolerance), and an adverse prognosis. The risk of hospitalization for decompensated heart failure and death is directly related to haemoglobin concentration. The predictive value of anaemia may reflect either an association with disease severity or be causally related to disease progression. Potential causal mechanisms include exacerbation of myocardial ischaemia, promotion of intravascular volume expansion, and increased neurohumoral activation. In support of this, the adverse prognosis conferred by anaemia appears to be independent of factors such as renal function and volume overload. Correction of anaemia using human recombinant erythropoietin with or without intravenous iron may improve symptoms, exercise capacity, and cardiac performance. However, results from large-scale double-blinded trials are needed to evaluate the efficacy and safety of this approach before it can be recommended as standard therapy.

Figure 10.3 Factors contributing to anaemia in CHF

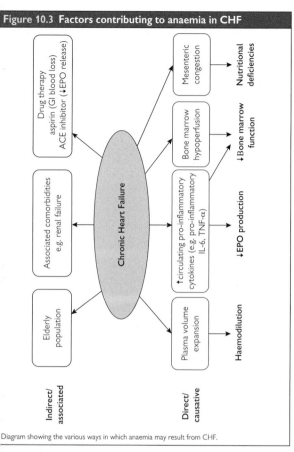

Diagram showing the various ways in which anaemia may result from CHF.

10.6 **Depression**

The prevalence of depression in patients with CHF ranges from 13% to 48% amongst outpatients and has been reported to be as high as 77% in hospitalised patients. Biological symptoms of depression such as fatigue, loss of libido, and poor appetite may be ascribed to heart failure or associated treatments and the condition frequently goes unrecognised and therefore untreated. Depression is associated with greater severity of physical symptoms (such as breathlessness and exercise limitation), more hospitalizations, and substantially higher healthcare costs than in patients without depression. The increased costs are not a reflection of mental-health utilization but rather directly attributable to heart-failure treatment. Furthermore most studies suggest coexistent depression in CHF is an independent risk factor for mortality. The reason for this excess of adverse outcomes is unclear but may involve reverse causation (i.e. the presence of more advanced disease may lead to depression) or poorer concordance with prescribed therapies. Suboptimal adherence to treatment is associated with greater mortality and morbidity in CHF and frequently accounts for hospitalizations with acute decompensated heart failure.

Although effective pharmacological and non-pharmacological treatments are available for the treatment of depression there have been no randomized trials in patients with heart failure. If pharmacological treatment is judged appropriate, selective serotonin reuptake inhibitors should probably be the agent of choice whilst tricyclic antidepressants are best avoided.

10.7 **Cognitive dysfunction**

Due to the greatly increased prevalence of heart failure in elderly patients there is, inevitably, an association between CHF and dementia. However, milder degrees of cognitive dysfunction are disproportionately common in patients with CHF compared with age-matched controls. This may, in part, reflect a greater risk of cerebrovascular events in patients with CHF, who have a high prevalence of atherosclerotic disease. Patients with CHF are also at greater risk of cardiogenic emboli as a result of associated atrial fibrillation and valvular disorders. An alternative (or complementary) explanation is that low cardiac output in CHF may lead to a degree of cerebral hypoperfusion. Interestingly studies of cardiac transplant recipients have demonstrated improved cognitive performance, suggesting that cognitive dysfunction may be at least partly reversible by increased cardiac performance.

At present, no interventions have been shown to improve cognitive dysfunction in patients with CHF. However, it is important to remember that co-existent depression is common in patients with CHF and may represent an underlying and treatable cause for cognitive impairment.

Key references

Braunstein, J.B., Anderson, G.F., Gerstenblith, G., *et al.* (2003). Noncardiac comorbidity increases preventable hospitalizations and mortality among Medicare beneficiaries with chronic heart failure. *J. Am. Coll. Cardiol.*, **42**, 1226–33.

Salpeter, S., Ormiston, T., Salpeter, E. (2005). Cardioselective beta-blockers for chronic obstructive pulmonary disease. *Cochrane Database Syst. Rev.*, **4**, CD003566.

Schiffrin, E.L., Lipman, M.L., Mann, J.F. (2007). Chronic kidney disease: effects on the cardiovascular system. *Circulation*, **116**, 85–97.

Felker, G.M., Adams, K.F. Jr., Gattis, W.A., O'Connor, C.M. (2004). Anemia as a risk factor and therapeutic target in heart failure. *J. Am. Coll. Cardiol.*, **44**, 959–66.

Konstam, V., Moser, D.K., De Jong, M.J. (2005). Depression and anxiety in heart failure. *J. Card. Fail.*, **11**, 455–63.

Chapter 11

Heart failure in the elderly

Nigel T. Lewis and Lip-Bun Tan

Key Points

- Ageing has profound effects on cardiovascular structure and function and predisposes individuals to development of chronic heart failure (CHF).
- In the UK, 89% of all CHF deaths and 74% of all CHF admissions occur in those individuals over 75 years of age.
- In older individuals CHF is more often multifactorial. CHF occurs when the heart's pumping capacity is impaired, either because of a structural, functional, or electrical abnormality of the heart.
- Multiple comorbidities and polypharmacy make elderly patients with CHF a particular challenge best approached using a multidisciplinary team approach.
- In many cases the emphasis may shift from extension of life expectancy to one of improving quality of life. End of life management issues should be borne in mind and palliative care.

11.1 Background

Chronic heart failure (CHF) is the cumulative effects of cardiological abnormalities that combine to result in functional impairment of the cardiac pumping ability. Not surprisingly, through passage of time, the older the patient, the greater the likelihood for the individual to have suffered one or more cardiac events culminating in the presentation of CHF. Of all the age groups the elderly have the highest incidence and prevalence of CHF. There are specific issues that are more relevant for this age group.

11.2 Common causes of Heart Failure in the elderly

In older individuals, CHF is more often multifactorial than it is in younger people. CHF occurs when the heart's pumping capacity is impaired, either because of a structural, functional or electrical abnormality of the heart. In addition it can be caused by ischaemic, metabolic, endocrine, infective, inflammatory, and neoplastic processes. Hypertension and coronary artery disease account for the majority of cases of CHF at older age. Hypertension is the leading cause in older women, accounting for 59% of cases and in older men coronary artery disease is the leading cause accounting for 39% of cases. This is followed by valvular heart disease non-ischaemic cardiomyopathy, and diabetes.

11.3 **Precipitating factors**

Establishing factors that precipitate or contribute to CHF exacerbations are equally important. Common factors include non-adherence with medication and fluid balance adjustments, myocardial infarction or ischaemia, arrhythmias (commonly atrial fibrillation or atrial flutter), renal dysfunction, chest infection, sepsis, anaemia, thyroid disease, adverse new pharmacotherapy (e.g. NSAIDs, dihydropyridines, thiazolidinediones), and excess alcohol consumption.

11.4 **Effects of ageing**

Ageing itself also produces profound effects on cardiovascular structure and function (see Box 11.1) and predisposes individuals to the development of CHF.

> ### Box 11.1 Effects of ageing on the cardiovascular system
>
> - Cumulative attrition of cardiomyocytes (gender differences)
> - Compensatory myocyte hypertrophy, causing eccentric left-ventricular hypertrophy, resulting in increased wall thickness with normal cavity size
> - Increased vascular hypertrophy and stiffness with increased impedance to left-ventricular ejection
> - Impaired endothelial function
> - Impaired left-ventricular diastolic filling
> - Impaired sinoatrial function and heart-rate variability
> - Reduced peak oxygen consumption
> - Reduced peak cardiac power output in men, but not women
> - Reduction in the aerobic enzyme activity of skeletal muscle, and thus a reduced peripheral oxygen extraction and ATP production capacity
> - Declining glomerular filtration rate

11.5 **Presentation**

Elderly patients often present with CHF in atypical ways and may be confounded or obscured by pre-existing comorbidities. As in younger adults, exertional dyspnoea, orthopnoea, and lower extremity swelling are common symptoms. However, many elderly patients attribute dyspnoea or exertional fatigue to the ageing process and often avoid orthopnoea by sleeping upright or in their chairs. Lower extremity swelling is common, but is non-specific because of multiple alternative causes in the elderly, including chronic venous insufficiency, chronic cellulites and ulceration, hepatic or renal dysfunction, and medication side effects.

More often elderly people present with atypical symptoms, such as confusion, irritability, somnolence, anorexia, oliguria, chest infection, and diminished activity ("off legs"). Therefore a higher index of suspicion is needed for diagnosing heart failure in elderly patients who are generally unwell.

Physical signs are similar to CHF presentation in younger patients, commonly with features of congestion, but it is important also to identify low output states leading to organ hypoperfusion. The latter may present with atypical features including, as discussed in Chapter 10, cognitive impairment, listlessness, and altered consciousness in the elderly.

11.6 **Diagnosis and investigations**

Determining the diagnosis of CHF in the elderly involves three necessary components: (i) the presence/absence of CHF; (ii) the cause(s) of CHF; (iii) the severity of CHF. As discussed in Chapter 3, objective tests are available to help clarify each of these diagnostic steps.

11.7 **Comorbidities**

As discussed in Chapter 10, conditions associated with higher risk of CHF hospitalizations and mortality include COPD, renal failure, diabetes, depression, and lower respiratory diseases. Reasons why elderly heart-failure patients have more adverse events could be because of lack of adherence to treatment. There are higher rates of non-compliance with therapy and failure of patients to understand their condition and seek assistance with symptom recurrence and also patients on multiple drugs ("poly-pharmacy") are susceptible to drug interactions.

11.8 **Therapeutic approaches**

The overall objectives of treatment for elderly patients with CHF are primarily to improve the quality of life and to improve longevity, although the latter is not necessarily of paramount importance if quality of life is poor.

The cornerstone of therapy involves identification and treatment of the underlying aetiology and precipitating factors. Although it is not always possible, a diligent search for reversible causes is important, as treatment often delays progression and improves symptoms; and if successful correction is achievable, this may even render the patient free from CHF. Precipitant factors like atrial fibrillation should be controlled by restoration to sinus rhythm or optimal rate control and anticoagulated appropriately depending on risk. Symptomatic brady-arrythmias should be paced, if they do not improve with stopping rate controlling medications. Anaemia should be corrected by supplementary iron or blood transfusions. Thyroid disease should be identified and corrected. Alcohol should be limited or ceased. Certain drugs should be avoided if at all possible, including non-steroidal anti-inflammatory drugs, steroids, cyclizine, and certain anti-depressant and antipsychotic drugs. Probably most importantly, adherence to prescribed medication and fluid-balance control should be emphasised and supervised.

Most clinical trials on the management of CHF have excluded individuals who were older than 75–80 years, and conducted in younger individuals. The main emphasis from these positive trials has been to improve prognosis and has not necessarily been accompanied by symptomatic or functional improvements. Therefore, it is important to distinguish which therapeutic agents are primarily for prognostic benefits and which for symptomatic or functional benefits.

11.8.1 **Pharmacotherapy**

For prognostic benefit

Angiotensin converting enzyme inhibitors, angiotensin receptor blockers, beta-blockers, and aldosterone antagonists reduce mortality in those with reduced ejection fractions. Low doses of these drugs should be used initially in elderly patients, as they are particularly at risk of hypotension and worsening renal impairment, and regular follow-up should be organised to monitor their progress during the initiation period.

For symptomatic benefit

Diuretics are still accepted as the first-line therapy for patients with CHF, despite the lack of large-scale randomized controlled trials. The main reason why diuretics are necessary is because a fundamental compensatory mechanism in CHF is to trigger retention of fluid. They are effective at relieving pulmonary and systemic congestion and maintaining euvolaemia. A crucial principle of diuretic therapy is that the doses should always be reactive to the extents of congestion (i.e. never to allow overdosage resulting in dehydration—resulting in renal impairment or the patient having to drink more to catch up with excess fluid loss). Patients need close monitoring of their electrolytes and renal function, as they are prone to hyponatraemia, hypokalaemia, and dehydration.

Venodilators, such as nitrates, are helpful in relieving the symptoms of venous congestions, complementing the effects of diuretics. Arterial vasodilators, such hydralazine, are particularly helpful in patients who are still relatively hypertensive, but the lowering of arterial pressure needs to be gradual to avoid symptoms of dizziness. Most vasodilators are combined venous and arterial vasodilators, and they may also improve symptoms. However, in most patients with advanced CHF, their arterial pressures are usually low, and they may have very little reserve to tolerate much arterial vasodilatation. Symptoms may therefore improve with a low dose vasodilator therapy but paradoxically worsen with larger doses.

11.8.2 Device therapy

Cardiac resynchronization therapy

As discussed ventricular conduction abnormality is associated with ventricular dysfunction and is reported in about 30% of CHF patients. Cardiac resynchronization therapy is a useful therapy in selected patients with benefit to ventricular function, exercise tolerance, and prognosis; although there are no prospective trials in the elderly. Therefore use in older patients must be individualised until further evidence becomes available.

Internal cardioveter-defibrillator

Although the internal cardioverter defibrillator can prevent arrhythmic death, it does not prevent death itself. Having the device in place can certainly affect the 'quality of death'. As heart failure or other comorbid disease progresses, it becomes important to address end-of-life issues and this would require the possibility of deactivation of the inernal cardioverter defibrillator. For these reasons many older patients are not offered these implants.

11.8.3 Multidisciplinary care

Multidisciplinary care is becoming increasingly important in the management of patients with CHF, it is especially important in management of elderly patients because of the multiple comorbidities, polypharmacy, and increased social care needed due to immobility or cognitive impairment. This involves close links with heart-failure specialist nurses, pharmacists, social workers, general practitioners, and cardiologists. Specific goals are to improve patients' education, compliance with medications, diet, and exercise and monitor patients' conditions in the community.

Withdrawal of treatment

It is advisable to address end of life issues, including resuscitation and withdrawal of medications, at an appropriate stage of CHF care and reconsider these issues as the disease progresses. The primary objective of management is to relieve symptoms, minimise discomfort and suffering, and withdraw therapies, which unintentionally delay death.

The principles of continuation or withdrawal of medication for end-stage CHF patients consist of the following:

- Drugs primarily prescribed to improve prognosis but also worsening symptoms or function should be withdrawn.
- Drugs primarily to improve symptoms, well-being, or function (e.g. diuretics, digoxin, vasodilators), irrespective of whether they improve prognosis or not, should be continued.
- Always use the lowest doses of drugs necessary to produce the desired symptomatic benefits, discarding the concept of aiming for 'trial-proven doses'.
- The frequency and doses of drugs should be given to cover sufficient durations. Inadequate regimens resulting in frequent break-through of symptoms can interrupt restful sleep and be quite distressing.

The last few days of life are accompanied frequently by considerable discomfort and anxiety and a cardinal principle is to provide adequate relief of dyspnoea, pain, and suffering through appropriate use of narcotics (morphine), sedatives (benzodiazepines), and other comfort measures. Equally important is to negotiate a place to die (home, hospice, or hospital) and to provide emotional and spiritual support for the patient and family, assisted by nurses and other health-care professionals.

11.9 Conclusions

CHF is a common disorder in elderly people and represents a challenge to health-care professionals. The involvement of a multidisciplinary team approach is invaluable and improves quality of life in elderly patients. Multiple pathologies may coexist and the emphasis in treatment often needs to shift from quantity to quality of life.

Key references

Wei, J.Y. (1992). Age and the cardiovascular system. *N. Engl. J. Med.*, **327**, 1735–9.

Olivetti, G., Melissari, M., Capasso, J.M., Anversa, P. (1991). Cardiomyopathy of the aging human heart. Myocyte loss and reactive cellular hypertrophy. *Circ. Res.*, **68**, 1560–8.

Ahmed, A., Allman, R.M., Aronow, W.S., DeLong, J.F. (2004). Diagnosis of heart failure in older adults: predictive value of dyspnea at rest. *Arch. Gerontol. Geriatr.*, **38**, 297–307.

Williams, S.G., Cooke, G.A., Wright, D.J., *et al.* (2001). Peak exercise cardiac power output; a direct indicator of cardiac function strongly predictive of prognosis in chronic heart failure. *Eur. Heart J.*, **22**, 1496–503.

Flather, M.D., Shibata, M.C., Coats, A.J., *et al.* (2005). Randomized trial to determine the effect of nebivolol on mortality and cardiovascular hospital admission in elderly patients with heart failure (SENIORS). *Eur. Heart J.*, **26**, 215–25.

Rich, M.W. (2006). Heart failure in older adults. *Med. Clin. North Am.*, **90**, 863–85.

Chapter 12

Advanced heart failure

Narbeh Melikian, Robin Ray, and
Mark Vanderheyden

Key Points

- Advanced heart failure, despite modern pharmacological therapies, has a poor prognosis.
- The management of patients with advanced heart failure needs a multidisciplinary approach involving specialist surgeons and physicians.
- A number of surgical approaches may improve outcomes in selected patients.
- Cardiac transplantation remains the definitive therapeutic approach for patients with advanced heart failure refractory to conventional treatments.
- If patients are unsuitable for these treatments therapeutic approaches may then switch to symptom control and quality-of-life or end-of-life issues.

12.1 Background

Despite major advances in the pharmacological management of chronic heart failure (using a combination of agents such as beta-blockers, angiotensin-converting-enzyme inhibitors, angiotensin-II-receptor antagonists, and diuretics), patients with advanced heart failure remain highly symptomatic with a poor prognosis. Over the past two decades a number of non-pharmacological interventions have been developed to manage patients with advanced heart failure. These therapies fall into four categories:

1. Complex pacing to achieve cardiac resynchronization using a biventricular pacemaker
2. Novel surgical techniques
3. Ventricular assist devices
4. Cardiac transplantation

Complex pacing has been discussed in detail in Chapter 7. This chapter will therefore focus on novel surgical techniques, ventricular assist devices, and cardiac transplantation.

12.2 **Surgical techniques**

A number of conventional and novel surgical approaches are available for management of patients with advanced or refractory heart failure.

12.2.1 **Conventional surgical techniques**

Coronary artery bypass surgery (CABG) and heart valve surgery are important tools in management of heart failure patients.

CABG

If pharmacological and device based therapeutic options are unsuccessful and other therapeutic approaches are needed patients with ischaemic cardiomyopathy should undergo non-invasive function testing (using echocardiography, MRI, PET, or both) to look for evidence of myocardial viability as opposed to scar tissue. All viable myocardium may then be revascularised (by use of PCI, CABG, or both), which may optimise myocardial contractile function.

Valve surgery

As with CABG, valve abnormalities can be corrected surgically to help reduce cardiac workload in the failing ventricle. The utility of repairing the dysfunctional mitral valve occurring as a result of left-ventricular dilatation at the moment remains unclear. However, it warrants consideration and application in selected patients.

12.2.2 **Novel surgical techniques**

Over the past two decades a number of non-coronary and non-valve surgical techniques for the management of advanced heart failure have been developed. However, no one procedure has provided consistent clinical improvement in heart-failure patients. Clinical outcomes from reports are highly variable and confined to small case series. The clinical utility of these techniques remains under question and their use is confined to individual patients in selected centres.

Dor procedure

Large left-ventricle aneurysms have a paradoxical motion in relation to the functional myocardium. This action increases the workload of the functional myocardium as it strives to maintain forward blood flow. The Dor procedure involves resection of the aneurysmal segment and bridging of the gap with an endoventricular patch to restore conical left-ventricle shape and a reduction in paradoxical motion. In patients with aneurysm-related left-ventricular failure, this procedure has been shown to be highly effective in improving symptoms with a mortality of around 7%.

Batista procedure (partial left ventriculectomy)

This procedure is based on the presumption that a reduction in left-ventricle radius will reduce wall stress (Laplace's law, see Chapter 2 for details) and hence improve systolic function. The surgical procedure involves partial removal of left-ventricle wall segments to reduce left-ventricle radius. However, clinical results remain disappointing and inconsistent with high mortality rates (up to 40% in some series).

Cardiomyoplasty

This technique involves wrapping of a skeletal muscle (commonly latissimus dorsi) around the left ventricle. There is some evidence that chronically stimulated skeletal muscle may convert into fatigue resistant type I fibres. However, clinical results have been poor with some series reporting improvements no better than optimal medical therapy.

ACORN cardiac support device

There is evidence that passive diastolic constraint of the left ventricle in heart-failure patients may prevent increasing diastolic left-ventricle filling and thus dilatation. Preventing left-ventricle dilatation may stabilise further deterioration of left-ventricular function and heart-failure symptoms. A biocompatible mesh (the ACORN device) is now available that can be fitted surgically over both ventricles (like a sock). Animal data have been encouraging, but human data are confined to a single case series, which demonstrated short-term improvement in symptoms. There are ongoing trials to investigate this technique further.

12.3 **Ventricular assist devices**

Ventricular assist devices can be used as a bridge to either recovery or cardiac transplantation in individuals with advanced heart failure in which other therapies have failed (see Figure 12.1). Clinical and haemodynamic indications for such devices are summarised in Box 12.1. Although most patients requiring a vascular assist device will be in cardiogenic shock (haemodynamic parameters outlined below), a final decision regarding the suitability of an individual patient for such a device is made jointly by cardiac surgical and cardiology teams.

Complications associated with prolonged use of vascular assist devices include:

- fulminant ventricular arrhythmias;
- hepatic or renal dysfunction;
- right heart failure;
- coagulopathy and bleeding;
- sepsis.

Valvular pathology may complicate insertion of vascular assist devices. Patients with aortic-valve stenosis and regurgitation and mitral valve stenosis will tolerate a vascular assist device poorly. It is recommended that these abnormalities are corrected surgically at the time of insertion. However, mitral valve regurgitation does not cause haemodynamic compromise with vascular assist device and can be left uncorrected.

12.5 Cardiac transplantation

12.5.1 Background

Heart transplantation is an accepted mode of treatment for patients with advanced heart failure in whom all other pharmacological, device, and surgical procedures have failed. The cornerstone of successful of transplantation remains effective and controlled immunosuppressive therapy, with the advent of such pharmacological agents in the 1980s paving the way for a major worldwide expansion in heart transplantation. There are currently around 300 cardiac transplant centres throughout the world and it was estimated that by the year 2000 a cumulative total of over 48,000 cardiac transplants had been performed. However, shortage of organ donors and eventual graft rejection remain major limitations of cardiac transplantation.

> **Box 12.1 Clinical and haemodynamic indications for insertion of vascular assist devices**
>
> *Clinical indications*
> 1. Acute cardiogenic shock in the context of:
>   —acute myocardial infarction;
>   —acute myocardtitis;
>   —severe left-ventricular dysfunction secondary to inherited or acquired cardiomyopathy;
>   —or patients unable to come off cardio-pulmonary bypass
> 2. Chronic heart failure patients on transplant waiting list who deteriorate acutely
> 3. Refractory malignant cardiac arrhythmia (such as ventricular tachycardia (VT) or ventricular fibrillation (VF))
> 4. Any other acute or chronic condition leading to severe left-ventricular dysfunction or cardiogenic shock, in which either recovery or transplantation could be a possibility
>
> *Haemodynamic parameters*
> 1. Cardiac index less than 2 L/min/m^2
> 2. Persistent systolic blood pressure less than 80 mm Hg
> 3. Capillary wedge pressure greater than 20 mm Hg

The indications for cardiac transplantation have remained stable over the years with the majority of transplants being performed for coronary artery disease and cardiomyopathy (see Box 12.2).

12.5.2 **Selection and exclusion criteria for cardiac transplantation and organ donors**

Strict guidelines govern both selection and exclusion of candidates for cardiac transplantation and organ harvesting.

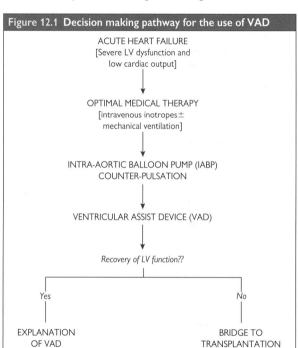

Figure 12.1 Decision making pathway for the use of VAD

ACUTE HEART FAILURE
[Severe LV dysfunction and
low cardiac output]

↓

OPTIMAL MEDICAL THERAPY
[intravenous inotropes ±
mechanical ventilation]

↓

INTRA-AORTIC BALLOON PUMP (IABP)
COUNTER-PULSATION

↓

VENTRICULAR ASSIST DEVICE (VAD)

↓

Recovery of LV function??

Yes   *No*

EXPLANATION   BRIDGE TO
OF VAD   TRANSPLANTATION

121

Box 12.2 Indications for cardiac transplantation

Coronary artery disease (45%)
Cardiomyopathies (45%)
Congenital heart disease (2%)
Valvular heart disease (4%)
Retransplantation (2%)
Miscellaneous causes (2%)

Selection of organ recipients

Typical candidates for cardiac transplantation have end-stage heart failure with less than 1 year estimated survival. A series of empirical criteria for acceptance and rejection of potential recipients exist. These criteria have been formulated to include patients with the greatest need for transplantation and to exclude individuals with conditions that may increase perioperative risk or decrease long-term survival (see Box 12.3).

12.5.3 **Organ allocation**

Donors and recipients require ABO blood-type compatibility and matching of body habitus. Prospective HLA matching is often not required. However, recipients often undergo panel reactive antibody screening. Only patients with greater than 20% panel positivity will require full prospective HLA crossmatch prior to transplantation.

Each cardiac centre is part of a computerised regional, national, and international registry of organ recipients and donors. Details on ABO blood type, body habitus, priority status, and geographic location of recipients are kept on these registries. As donor organs become available, cardiac transplant coordinators allocate matched organs to the highest priority cases initially on a regional then national basis. In the absence of suitable national recipients organs are offered internationally.

12.5.4 **Post-transplant management**

Management of heart transplant patients immediately postoperatively is beyond the scope of this book. We will therefore discuss the long-term management of these patients. Effective and controlled immunosuppressive therapy directed towards preventing organ rejection and complications of immunosuppression (such as infections and malignancy) are vital. Other complications include accelerated atherosclerosis and donor-heart failure.

Allograft rejection and maintenance of immunosuppression

There is no standard immunosuppressive therapy regime. However, most cardiac centres use triple immunosuppression therapy with prednisolone, ciclosporin and azathioprine or mycophenolate mofetil (MMF) or both as first-line therapy. In some centres, steroid therapy may start prior to transplantation and is often withdrawn rapidly to prevent complications. Percutaneous endomyocardial biopsy remains the gold standard for detection of allograft rejection. Each cardiac centre will have its own biopsy protocol. In general, patients are monitored very closely in the initial most vulnerable phase (months 1–3), with gradual reduction in the frequency of biopsies over a period of 12–18 months.

Escalation of immunosuppressive therapy is needed in patients in whom biopsy samples demonstrate evidence of rejection. Most centres use pulses of steroids as fist-line treatment of rejection. In patients with persistent rejection, photophoresis, total lymphoid irradiation, and re-transplantation are considered.

Box 12.3 Criteria used for selection and rejection of cardiac transplant recipients

Selection criteria for potential cardiac transplant patients

1. End-stage heart failure patients unresponsive to all other pharmacological and device therapy with a life expectancy of less than 1 year. Often these candidates have been inpatients for prolonged periods with the following:
   —Prolonged mechanical circulatory support
   —Ventilator-dependent heart failure
   —Continuous infusion of inotropic agents
   —Life expectancy of less than 7 days
2. Inoperable coronary artery disease with intractable angina symptoms
3. Malignant ventricular arrhythmias unresponsive to both medical and surgical therapy

Contraindications for cardiac transplantation

1. Age greater than 65 years
2. Severe pulmonary hypertension
3. Recent (past 6–8 weeks) history of pulmonary infarction
4. Evidence of significant end-organ damage due to diabetes
5. Any chronic illness affecting survival or function status
6. Symptomatic or severe peripheral vascular and carotid disease
7. Active infection
8. Severe, chronic or irreversible functional damage to any vital organ (including renal, pulmonary, hepatic failure)
9. Severe obesity (greater than 130% ideal body weight) or cachexia (less than 80% ideal body weight)
10. Drug, alcohol, or tobacco abuse in the previous 6 months
11. Psychiatric illness or poor medical compliance
12. Active or recent malignancy
13. HIV infection

Infection

Reduced cellular immunity exposes cardiac transplant patients to a wide range of infections with typical and atypical organisms. Infections must be treated aggressively. This is often achieved as a team effort between transplant physicians and surgeons, infectious disease specialists, and microbiologists.

Accelerated transplant atherosclerosis

Immune and non-immune injury to the endothelium leads to a unique accelerated form of coronary artery disease with an incidence of 10% per annum. Treatment options are the same as for non-transplant patients including percutaneous coronary intervention and CABG surgery. Accelerated transplant atherosclerosis is a major cause of death after transplantation.

12.5.5 Quality of life and prognosis

Quality of life is generally very good. Most patients are able to return to work. However, exercise capacity is reduced by 30–40% in comparison to normal individuals secondary to donor–recipient mismatch leading to restrictive physiology, chronotropic incompetence in the denervated donor heart, residual respiratory muscle, or systemic-muscle abnormalities that may persist post-transplantation or as a result of immunosuppressive therapy. First year survival for cardiac transplant patients is now over 80%. Of those who survive the first year, over 50% will be alive by 11 years.

12.6 Palliative care

If all therapeutic options have been explored and used or discounted then patients with advanced chronic heart failure represent an important challenge in terms of end-of-life issues. Cardiologists are often poor at changing their mindset to one of doing less to a patient. However, success in management of patients with advanced chronic heart failure can be judged in a number of ways. A death that is planned with a patient and relatives with palliative-care input is often a much better outcome than repeated hospitalizations for intravenous inotropes and diuretics. Very advanced chronic heart failure therefore needs specialist input from a palliative-care specialist who should be an integral part of the multidisciplinary team (see Chapter 11)

12.7 Summary

Advanced heart failure is a common disorder and requires a careful multidisciplinary approach including physician, surgeon, imaging specialists and specialist nurses. A number of options are available with the gold standard proven therapy being orthotopic cardiac transplantation. For non-transplant centres developing a dynamic good relationship with the transplant centre is important. If a patient is unsuitable for these more advanced therapies a decision should then be made regarding how aggressive therapies should be.

Key references

Stevenson, L.W., Rose, E.A. (2003). Left ventricular assist devices. Bridges to transplantation, recovery, and destination for whom? *Circulation*, **108**, 3059–63.

Alert, N.M., Davis, M., Young, J. (2002). Improving the care of patients dying of heart failure. *Clevland Clin. J. Med.*, **69**, 321–8.

Johnson, M.J. (2007). Management of end stage cardiac failure. *Postgrad. Med. J.*, **83**, 395–401.

Costanzo, M., Augustine, S., Bourge, R., *et al.* (1995). Selection and treatment of candidates for heart transplantation. *Circulation*, **92**, 3593–612.

Fang, J.C., Couper, G.S. (2002). 'Circulatory support devices', in Antman, E.M. (ed.), *Cardiovascular therapeutics. A Companion to Braunwald's Heart Disease*, 2nd edn. WB Saunders, Philadelphia, 1180–4.

NICE (2007). Heart failure—cardiac resynchronization, www.nice.org.uk/TA120, 2007.

Index

Contents

Contents

1

Indians Today

For the last two decades the subject of race relations in America has dominated our concern. Beginning before the early Civil Rights movement and continuing until the present many people, particularly church people, have been determined to bring a higher sense of justice into the relationships between groups of people. It should be no surprise, therefore, that American Indians should receive attention.

The mythology of the American Indian has long stood in the way of a more profound understanding of where Indians fit into the general American scheme of things. In the days when the "melting pot" theory was popularly expounded as the explanation of American social dynamics, Indians were seen as a vanishing group that had to give up their traditional ways and become "Indian Americans." Today many people still insist on calling Indians "Indian Americans" because the term symbolizes to them the unity which they hope will one day come about in our country.

"Indian Americans" is not a welcome name in Indian circles, however, since the name implies a general blurring of issues and an assumption that the strong tribal traditions have no ultimate reality in themselves. Just what "Indians" are to be called today remains a subject of great debate. Anthropologists have attempted to call us "Amerindians" or "Amerinds," but the phrase has not caught on. A great many younger Indian people have tried to popularize the phrase "Native Americans," but the older generation feels ill at ease with this name. In all probability no name other than "Indians" will ever satisfy most of the people known popularly as "Indians."

Hundreds of books trace the early history and culture of the respective tribes. Indeed, the subject of the Indian wars, from 1862-1890, must be one of the most frequently covered subjects in all of publishing. Dee Brown was not the first writer to tell the story of those years, but may have been the best and most sympathetic of those who did. We shall not deal with tribal histories or Indian wars, including Wounded Knee I, in this book. Rather, we shall deal with some aspects now coming into view that give a different perspective to the problems of American Indians today.

One of the most intriguing aspects of Indian life today is the manner in which the past continues to dominate the present and future. Most of the protests and struggles of the last five years have dealt with the violation of treaties or with efforts to get tribal lands restored to the tribes. In developing the arguments used to support the Alaska Native Land Claims legislation, or to justify the restoration of Blue Lake to the people of Taos Pueblo in New Mexico, or to get the Menominees treaty rights restored to them, we have seen the beginning of a new field of understanding. That field combines history and law and could be called historical law or legal history, depending on which subject receives more stress from the writer and which receives more interest from the reader.

It is through the device of historical law that we shall try to understand the situation of American Indians today. Through historical law we shall come to understand the background of the modern Indian movement and try to project where that movement is going and what can be done to make it more effective.

There are some American Indians in each state of the union, including Hawaii. Not all of them are living on their traditional lands. In fact, a great many of the Indians in the United States today are living far from the places that their ancestors originally inhabited. At least a part of the current protest involves the history of how the different groups of Indians came to live where they are now.

The census of 1970 showed that about 763,594 Indians live in the United States today. Of that number 70 percent live off their reservations and half live in small towns and cities. This figure is in sharp contrast to previous censuses which showed a majority of the Indians living on their reservations or within a short distance of them. One major reason why so many Indians live off their reservations is that nearly twenty years ago the United States government began a program called Relocation. Its purpose was to move as many Indians to the large cities as possible with the hope that they would be assimilated into the urban population and disappear.

Relocation operated in this fashion. An employee of the Bureau of Indian Affairs, the government agency with responsibility for providing services to Indians living on the reservations, would visit an Indian home on the reservation and would talk with the family and paint a beautiful picture of how good it was to live in the city. He or she would then use every trick conceivable to convince the family that they should move to the city. The government, the agent would say, offered training in job skills, payment of rent and living expenses while they were learning a trade, and assistance in finding a home in the urban area where they were to be relocated.

The program sounded fine, but it didn't work. The families were brought to cities on the West Coast and in the Midwest and put into a training program. Since the purpose was to get as many Indians off the reservation as possible, the government tried to limit its assistance to families in the program and put them on their own quickly. A man who had been promised assistance in learning a trade found that, if he was offered a job of any kind while in training, the government bureaucrats would insist that he take it. Once he did, he would lose all support and would be expected to earn a living for himself and his family, even though the job did not pay enough to support a family in the city. The drop-out rate in this program was extremely high.

A number of other factors caused Indians to move back to the reservations. Some misguided people, including many church people who wanted to help Indians, insisted that the Indian families should not live in the same neighborhood. The theory was based on the experience of blacks who had gathered together in neighborhoods when they had come to the cities. The results were black ghettos. For this reason people who helped Indians find homes in the cities deliberately located houses geographically distant from each other in order to prevent the creation of an Indian ghetto.

The result of this housing pattern was to deny Indian families any significant contact with other Indians who might be living in the same city. Indian families were not used to living alone like the whites and other city groups. They were used to visiting their friends and relatives frequently, and when they discovered that they did not know anyone in the city, many simply packed their goods and departed for the reservations where they could enjoy a rich community life.

Employment discrimination was another factor that prevented many Indians from remaining in the cities. Indians were denied advancement in their jobs because it was the fashion then to deny all racial minorities a chance to be promoted. In addition, some aspects of Indian life worked against the Indians achieving a good employment record. Many Indians belonged to tribal societies and they had to return to their reservations for dances and ceremonies. Everybody understood missing work for Christmas and Fourth of July, but nobody seemed to understand missing work for the Sun Dance or the Annual Fair and Rodeo of the tribe.

The relocation program proved to be such a disaster that the Bureau of Indian Affairs was told not to push people into the program and it was renamed "Employment Assistance." It was the same old program and a change of name did not help much. Perhaps the only real effect of the relocation program was to keep the reservations in a constant state of turmoil, as families were broken up and tribal customs disrupted by people coming and going on relocation. At any rate, many Indian families did settle in the cities and produced the concentrations of Indians that we find in the urban areas today.

While nearly 70 percent of Indians today live off their reservations, a large percentage of the remaining Indians do not live on their ancestral homelands. During the 1830s the policy of the United States was to make the Indians living east of the Mississippi River move to Nebraska, Kansas and Oklahoma so that the whites living in the East could have their lands. Some of the tribes moved peaceably, but others were taken on forced death marches to the barren plains of the trans-Mississippi West. These lands were given to the Indians because the white people running the government saw no other use for them. The whites had been used to living in the forests and marking off their property lines with rail fences. In the plains country they found no trees and saw that it would be impossible to mark boundaries, so they gave the lands to the Indians. When the whites later discovered barbed wire and learned how to fence the plains, they promptly began to move the Indians to small reservations, particularly in Oklahoma.

At one time the federal government planned to concentrate all of the Indians in the United States in what is now Oklahoma, then called Indian Territory. The reasoning was to move all of the Indians out of the other states, thereby stopping the Indian wars. But when it came to moving very strong tribes, like the Apache and the Sioux, the government was not strong enough and the plan was dropped. Nearly sixty tribes from other parts of the country were finally brought to Oklahoma. The policy of concentrating the tribes in a few states became a determining factor in the development of present Indian communities.

By the time the Indian wars had ended, the

treaties between the government and the tribes had been violated in many ways. The Sioux had lost the Black Hills and the Pueblo's land had been reduced to very small pieces in New Mexico. The Apaches had been pursued through the deserts of the Southwest and even the friendly Apache scouts, who had helped the Army capture Geronimo, had been sent to Florida as prisoners of war. In 1887, when the government began dividing the large tracts of tribal lands into small allotments and purchasing the remainder for the cattlemen, the situation of many tribes was desperate.

The Nez Percé of Chief Joseph, for example, first had a reservation allotted to them in the Wallova Valley of Oregon. Then they were forced from that reservation and endured the famous flight to Canada. Following their capture, they were taken to Oklahoma and given a small tract of land. Many of them died and after a number of years the remnants of the band were taken to the new Colville Reservation in northeastern Washington state where they were left friendless and without rights among a people who had been their enemies.

The Cheyennes were taken south to western Oklahoma in 1877, the year after the Custer fight at the Little Bighorn. There they languished, dying in incredible numbers because of the poor climate and scanty rations. They were really mountain and high plains people and could not endure the desert-like atmosphere of western

Oklahoma. The Apaches, who were forced to leave mountain homelands of the Arizona plateau and move either to Florida or to the deserts of Arizona, also suffered greatly from the change in climate.

From 1887 to the middle 1920s the land on most of the reservations was allotted to individual Indians. Each was given from 80 to 160 acres, depending upon the condition and whether it was classified as farming or grazing land. Railroads received rights of way across the reservations because the government felt that having transportation facilities near the Indians would make them easier to control.

During this whole period the government worked very hard to undermine the power of the traditional chiefs. Government agents refused to deal with the traditional leaders, preferring to work only with those Indians who would obey their wishes. It was only during times of crisis, when a chief such as Joseph or Red Cloud could prevent violence by his prestige in the tribe, that the government dealt with real Indian leaders.

The Christian churches were given control of reservations because the government thought that they would be most effective in civilizing the Indians. Today most Indians have very hard feelings toward the churches for their activities among the tribes in the 1880s and 1890s. But in fairness the policy of giving the churches control over the reservations was not all bad. The Army, for example, was deferred from violence against the Indians by the presence of missionaries. Churches also provided the education of the Indian children on many reservations until the government developed its own schools decades later. While the church mission schools were intended primarily to convert the children to Christianity and to stamp out tribal culture and customs, the Indians educated in these schools served as the community leaders during the critical years of the 1920s and 1930s.

The conditions of Indians today have been largely determined by what happened during those early years. In 1906 the Colvilles had to surrender the northern half of their reservation, which was opened to settlement. Not all of the land was settled, so in the 1950s the tribe asked for its return. The Congress gave back the land with the provision that the tribe submit a plan to terminate all relationships with the U.S. within five years. The Colvilles fought this provision from 1958 to 1970 when Congress relented.

Similar events occurred with other tribes; it is fair to say that most of the current problems of Indians have resulted from the failure of the United States government to deal fairly with the tribes during the period 1880-1910. It is upon this stage that the events of recent times have been played. Few people understand how the past has affected the Indians and the tendency of recent years has been simply to lash out in the hope of making some changes for the better.

2
The Twentieth Century

The period of Indian history between 1890 and 1920 remains very cloudy and unclear. Most writers about Indians seemed to think that, with the slaughter of the Big Foot band of Minneconjou Sioux at Wounded Knee in 1876, Indians became a part of America's past and they were better left there. Unfortunately this attitude has prevailed until very recent times and has affected both Indians and non-Indians. Few people in the tribes today can give an accurate accounting of what happened to their tribes during this thirty-year period and the current effort to reclaim the glory of former days by reviving the traditions of a century ago does not reckon with the very real changes in both tribal customs and government policy that took place during those years.

By the mid-1890s most of the tribes were in the process of receiving allotments of land under the General Allotment Act passed in 1887. This act gave the President the authority to negotiate with the tribes for cession to the federal government of what came to be called "surplus lands." The lands were surplus in the sense that most tribes owned more than the 160 acres-per-tribal-member allotment. It was the intent of the several Presidents in office during that period to reduce the tribal land holdings to 160 acres-per-member.

The chief tool for achieving land cessions from the Indians was the agreement process. The President appointed a "chief Indian Commissioner" to visit the reservations and negotiate a cession of land from the tribe living there. The promises often revolved about the question of an immediate cash payment on a per capita basis to the tribal members. The Indian people had not yet become accustomed to the cash economy, and while able to support themselves by raising cattle, farming, fishing and hunting, they rarely had any hard cash to purchase the new food stuffs of the white man. Tobacco, flour, coffee, sugar and ammunition could not be produced on the reservations and the people were always in need of cash to purchase these supplies. It became a simple matter to get the tribal members to agree to a land cession, if the government representative promised that each member would get a cash payment of $100 when the transaction was completed.

This practice set a number of very bad precedents. The people looked at their land resources as a source of immediate cash and thereafter there were always some tribal members, remembering the government payments, who wanted to sell the reservations. During the 1950s, when the Congress was pushing the termination policy, the Klamath tribal members sold their forest lands at a greatly reduced price just to get money for immediate use. Throughout this century there has been an unrelenting fear among the reservation people that one day enough tribal members would be willing to sell the lands that the government would force the others to sell their share too, completely liquidating the tribe.

The allotment process also confused the people as to exactly who were tribal members. Under the various agreements those people who agreed to sell the surplus lands and take allotments were to be given full citizenship after twenty-five years. During this period the lands were to be held in a federal trust. In due time some of the allotments had their twenty-five year trust period expire and the allottees were held to be citizens. However, some of these remained in need of federal services, so the Secretary of the Interior, upon petition of the tribal elders, declared that the allotted lands were to remain in trust.

The reverse of this practice was also true. Even before the trust period had expired an Indian allottee could be declared competent by a Court of Competency. Whenever the federal government wanted to free some of the reservation allotments from its control for cattlepersons and farmers to purchase them, it would set up a Court of Competency and declare those Indians

competent who held prime lands. The Indians had
no choice but to sell their lands. Using this technique, the government took many acres of Indian
lands during the 1890s and 1900s.

Following the enactment of the General Allotment Act in 1887, the government proceeded on
the theory that the granting of individual lands
to the Indians would result in civilizing them
through the effects of private ownership of property. This belief was very strongly held by the
Christian churchmen who gave their support to
the allotment policy. The policy had hardly been
tested before a problem arose concerning the
management of the lands. Many allotments had
been given to children when the agreements
were signed and these children later spent years
in the government boarding schools. Bureau of
Indian Affairs agents found that the allotments
belonging to these Indian children had lain idle
and produced no income while the children were
away at school.

The federal policy was to interpret the trust
period as a time when the lands should produce
a set percentage of income, as if the lands were
an investment. Since the allotments of some Indian children had not produced any income, the
bureaucrats worried that the government would
incur liability for failing to fulfill its trust responsibility. So in 1891 the General Allotment Act was
amended to allow leasing of Indian allotments by
the local agent, if he found that the lands belonged to minors or adults who were incompe-

tent. This act may have been the single most destructive law ever passed in the field of Indian Affairs.

The law was no sooner passed than it was used to lease as much Indian land as possible. Not only Indian children had their lands leased, but almost any Indian who did not take care of his or her allotment. Sometimes the agent would insist on leasing the Indian allotment because he decided that the Indian was not making proper use of the land and that the local cattlepeople and farmers could produce a much better return. In short order the abuses were staggering. In 1916 the Oglala Sioux of the Pine Ridge Indian Reservation in South Dakota owned more than 2 million acres that they used for their cattle, with the exception of one forty-acre tract. The government agent was replaced and the new agent sold most of their cattle and leased almost 80 percent of the land to white cattlepersons, who then drove their own cattle upon the land. The Sioux have never been able to break this stranglehold and part of the demands at Wounded Knee in 1973 involved breaking these leases and returning the lands to the Sioux people.

The tribes of Oklahoma suffered the most from agreements and allotments. Originally these tribes had been omitted from the implementation of the General Allotment Act because they were making such good progress toward civilization. Senator Henry Dawes, after a visit to the Five Civilized Tribes (Cherokee, Choctaw, Chickasaw, Creek and Seminole), related his experiences to a meeting of philanthropists at Lake Mohonk, New York, in 1885:

> The head chief told us that there was not a family in that whole Nation that had not a home of its own. There was not a pauper in that Nation, and the Nation did not owe a dollar. It built its own capitol . . . and it built its schools and its hospitals. Yet the defect of the system was apparent. They have got as far as they can go, because they own their land in common. It is Henry George's system, and under that there is no enterprise to make your home any better than that of your neighbors. There is no selfishness, which is at the bottom of civilization. Till this people will consent to give up their lands, and divide them among their citizens so that each can own the land he cultivates, they will not make much more progress.

The Five Civilized Tribes used the assignment system. Any family could have as much land as they wanted, if they would promise to take care of it. The tribal government assigned them the lands they chose; if the family moved or stopped using the lands, they reverted to the tribe and other families could then apply for their use.

In these days of escalating poverty and national debt, it seems incredible that the federal government would deliberately destroy a system of government that had accomplished so much. But it did. The Five Civilized tribes had accepted many white persons on their lands; in the late 1880s these whites turned on their hosts and demanded that the government allot the lands of the Five Tribes to them. Since the proportion of whites to Indians was nearly four to one within the boundaries of the tribal lands, the government saw that it would be easy and popular to force allotment on the tribes.

In a series of swift moves the Congress stripped the governments of the Five Civilized Tribes of their governing powers and authorized the Dawes Commission to negotiate with the Oklahoma tribes for the sale of their surplus lands. The tribes refused to discuss allotment; so in 1895, Congress authorized a survey of their lands and the following year it directed the Dawes Commission to prepare rolls of the tribal members for eventual allotment. Still the tribes refused to negotiate; they had confirmed titles to their lands under the Removal Treaties of the 1830s and they demanded that the United States live up to its word. Finally in 1898, when all threats and bribes had failed, Congress passed the Curtis Act that simply allotted the lands of the Cherokees, Creeks, Choctaws, Chickasaws and Seminoles.

The governments of the Five Civilized Tribes were virtually abolished under the Curtis Act. The fine school system that had been developed by the tribes was merged into the government school system and allotments were handed out to the tribal members. Making the traditional members of the tribes accept their allotments was

easier said than done. They looked upon acceptance of an allotment as a violation of their treaties and they refused to touch the pen.

The traditional Indians in each of the tribes
tried to find ways of avoiding the implications of
the Curtis Act. The Choctaws petitioned Congress
to allow them to sell all of their lands and move
to South America. Jacob Jackson, a Choctaw full-
blood, gave the views of the traditional people
before a Senate committee in 1906:

> Surely a race of people, desiring to preserve the
> integrity of that race, who love it by reason of
> its traditions and their common ancestors and
> blood, who are proud of the fact that they be-
> long to it may be permitted to protect them-
> selves, if in no other way by emigration. Our
> educated people inform us that the white man
> came to this country to avoid conditions which
> to him were not as bad as the present conditions
> are to us. . . . All we ask is that we may be
> permitted to exercise the same privilege.

Congress, of course, rejected the plea of the
Choctaws and made them take allotments. The
surplus lands of the Oklahoma tribes became the
object of the great land rushes during the 1890s
and 1900s. When Oklahoma finally became a
state in 1907, by combining the former Oklahoma
Territory and the old Indian Territory, 1.4 million
people lived there, of whom only 75,000 were
descendants of the original Indian inhabitants.

By 1920 most of the reservations had been allotted. Government agents even came to the barren Hopi Reservation in central Arizona and tried to force the Hopi people to take allotments. Their land was so barren that they could farm only the small gulches between the mountains and mesas, yet the government, singlemindedly pursuing its policy, tried to pretend that the desert was tillable and therefore capable of being divided into agricultural allotments.

The story of the American Indian might have ended with the tribes slowly sinking into obscurity had it not been for a singular event. The Pueblo Indians of New Mexico had been classified as citizens for many years because of their former Mexican citizenship. By the 1848 Treaty of Guadalupe Hildalgo all citizens of the New Mexico territory were given the choice of remaining under American rule or migrating to Mexico. Those who chose to remain were to have their property rights upheld by the American government. From 1848 to 1912 the territorial courts of New Mexico systematically confiscated the lands of the Pueblos under a number of excuses and the federal government, fearing that it did not have jurisdiction over the Pueblos, stood by and allowed them to be dispossessed.

At the turn of the century the liquor trade among the Pueblos became a very serious matter and a number of suits was filed in an effort to determine whether or not the federal government could stop the trade in spirits in the Pueblo villages. In a landmark case, *United States v. Sando-*

val, the Supreme Court ruled that the United States government had full and total jurisdiction over the lands and lives of the Pueblos. The effect of the decision was to void all of the property titles to the lands that had been illegally taken from the Pueblos in the preceding half century.

The whites in New Mexico were livid and they recruited then Senator Hiram Bursum to clear their titles. Bursum introduced a bill in Congress which would have had the effect of making the Pueblo people prove that they owned their own lands. The bill had cleared the Senate and was being considered in the House before the Pueblos heard about it. Realizing they faced legal extinction the Pueblos called their All-Pueblo Council into session. It was the first time that all of the Pueblo villages had united since they drove the Spanish out of New Mexico in 1680.

The Pueblos were aided by the General Federation of Women's Clubs and several organizations interested in Indian affairs in forming a coalition to oppose the Bursum bill. John Collier, a small man who had formerly been a social worker in New York City, led the coalition in taking their case to the American public. The Bursum bill was stopped and in 1924 the Pueblos were able to get Congress to enact a much more favorable bill which required the white squatters to prove their land titles. A special attorney was assigned to the Pueblos under the law to institute ejectment suits; by the late 1930s over three thousand people had been ejected from the Pueblos' lands.

The fight over the Pueblo lands proved to be the turning point in the twentieth century for American Indians. All over the nation tribes watched the struggle of the Pueblos and took heart. No longer would they remain silent while their lands were despoiled; soon many tribes were contacting lawyers and making trips into the nation's capitol in search of justice. Collier founded the American Indian Defense Association and led a national fight to reverse the many bad policies that were being promoted by the career employees of the Bureau of Indian Affairs. Out of Collier's fight came a special report, the Meriam Report in 1928, that advocated a great many changes in the status of Indians and had great influence on the later actions of Congress.

Although there are many paths leading into the last century that explain the current problems of Indians, the most important changes and ideas discussed today are those triggered in the late 1920s and early 1930s and resulting directly from the Pueblos' successful fight against impossible odds.

3

Recent Reforms

The 1930s may seem a century away, but the events of that decade are still within the memory of many people today. The reforms of the 1930s are so important to understand the problems of Indians today that we begin our discussion of the modern era with what happened to American Indians during the New Deal. Within that context the events of Wounded Knee 1973 and take-over of Alcatraz will begin to make a great deal of sense.

The 1920s saw the beginning of a great movement for reform of the conditions of American Indians. The scandals of the Harding administration involved the distribution of mineral royalties due on Indian lands and, as the 1920s drew to a close, the attention of the American public began to focus on Indian problems much as it did forty years later. Unlike the sixties, the twenties were characterized by a number of studies that outlined the problems of Indians in a sensible man-

ner. The Meriam Report advocated a change in
federal Indian policy from its role as caretaker of
Indian lands to the role of educator of Indian
people. Not all of its recommendations were
carried out, but the general principles of reform
advocated by the report were accepted by Congress as sensible proposals.

The Senate Indian Committee rejected the
Meriam Report and decided to conduct its own
study; from 1928 to 1932 the Senate committee
toured the western reservations holding open
hearings on the conditions of Indians. The Senators were astounded to discover that the conditions of Indians all over the country were as
bad as the Meriam Report had indicated. Every-
where the committee members went they found
evidence of government mismanagement of Indian lands and resources and a deteriorating situation compounded by a lack of direction in the
government policies. Tribe after tribe appeared
before the committee to curse the allotment program as the cause of their extreme poverty.
Many tribes asked the government to investigate
the violations of their treaties, remarking that
they had been denied the right to sue the United
States for its misuse of their lands and funds.

Congress was in the mood for some radical
change by 1932 and the incoming New Deal
Congress proved to be the ideal vehicle to promote that change. The administration of Franklin
Roosevelt turned the Bureau of Indian Affairs
upside down and reversed the old processes of

decay. John Collier, the reformer who had helped the Pueblos defeat the Bursum Bill, was named Commissioner of Indian Affairs and he drew up a new program designed to emphasize the strengths of the old tribal traditions. His program was called the Indian Reorganization Act and he visualized building a new type of Indian community by giving the tribes self-government, thus relieving the federal bureaucracy of its power over the reservations.

A cornerstone of Collier's new program was to give to the reservations a corporate charter, a constitution and bylaws for the government of the tribes. The people on each reservation would be free to accept or reject the new law; if they accepted it, they would be exempted from further allotments, their present lands would remain in an indefinite federal trust, and they would be given federal loans for economic development of their resources. Collier hoped that the old tribal solidarity would reassert itself and he included a provision that all existing allotments of land would be kept in tribal ownership in the pending legislation.

This return to tribal ownership provision proved to be Collier's undoing. Many of the Indians had kept their allotments in trust and refused to cede them back to tribal ownership. They foresaw the day when the federal government might again demand allotments and decided that they would be more likely to retain their land through individual ownership. Many of them also were angry that those Indians who had sold their lands would receive the benefits of tribal lands, if the allotments were given back to the tribe. So adamant were the landowners that Collier was forced to scrap his land consolidation plan; when the final version of Collier's program passed the Congress it had few of the beneficial provisions that he had originally planned.

The defeat of Collier's efforts at reform had little immediate impact. It was not until Wounded Knee 1973 that many people began to understand how drastic the changes in the Indian Reorganization Act had been. In 1934 and 1935 the people from the Bureau of Indian Affairs had included many Indians who had already left the tribes in the vote on the Indian Reorganization Act. Very few of the tribes had up to date rolls, and in their enthusiasm to get the reservations to accept the I.R.A., Bureau employees did everything possible to get the Indians to vote "yes" on the act.

The traditional people on many of the reservations did not want the new form of government under the Indian Reorganization Act, so they refused to vote on the proposal. The Bureau, in order to get the act passed, allowed disenfranchised Indians to vote. The result was that on many reservations a constitution and bylaws were adopted, but the people running the new government were not those who owned the lands of the reservations. More often they were people who had already sold their lands and remained in the agency towns seeking part-time work, or living as best they could on relief when there was no work. The tribal governments created under the I.R.A. had to pay more attention to these non-owners because of their many votes than they did to the traditional people who had held onto their lands.

Soon two forms of government appeared on some of the reservations. The traditional people continued to exercise whatever control they could over the outlying villages and settlements of the reservations, while the new tribal officials recognized by the federal government tried to govern the reservations under the new law. Mixed into the new experiment were all the old abuses that had occurred under the Bureau of Indian Affairs. The cattlepeople still controlled the grazing lands, but now they had to become friends with both the Bureau of Indian Affairs employees *and* the tribal officials. The cattlepeople invested a great deal of money in the tribal elections because the tribal councils had the right and power to determine the grazing and farming policies of the reservations. Antagonisms between the two groups of Indians began to grow.

The Second World War was instrumental in stopping the operations of the Indian Reorganization Act on the reservations. No funds were available for development of the reservation lands because everything had to be devoted to winning the war. New plans developed by the tribal councils were never carried out and much of the progress achieved in the late thirties was wasted because projects were never finished.

With peace came a determination to fulfill the American dream. Many Americans thought it ridiculous to proclaim that the war had been fought to keep people free while black citizens in the United States were not treated as well as the German and Italian prisoners of war. The reason for the disparity, of course, was racial prejudice, but the sentiment for reform of domestic America had begun to grow. The National Council of Churches did a study of Indian conditions, but failing to understand the history of Indians, saw in the existence of the reservations only a perpetuation of segregation. The Council concluded that abolishment of the reservations should be the proper federal policy.

The churches had been traditionally allies with the Indians and, even though they had supported the General Allotment Act in 1887, they had supported the Pueblos and other peoples in their struggles in the intervening decades. Suddenly the churches and the conservative congressmen were on the same side, and with no visible allies, the Indians were vulnerable to a change of policy from the self-government of the New Deal to the termination of treaty rights. In 1954 this policy was put into effect and nineteen tribes lost federal recognition. Dozens more were threatened with the loss of their treaty rights before an Indian coalition, led by the National Congress of American Indians, put a stop to it.

The Klamaths of Oregon, the Menominees of Wisconsin, the Mixed Blood Utes of Utah and a number of smaller tribes lost federal services and supervision during the height of the termination policy. By late 1956 the Indian tribes had been aroused and they exhibited their discontent at the polls. Indian voting strength scared many a Senator and Congressman representing the western states and unseated one anti-Indian Congressman in Montana. By 1958 the Secretary of the Interior announced that no other tribes would be pressured to terminate their federal relationship. Although the Senate Interior Committee compelled the Colville tribe to prepare a termination plan in order to get their lands restored to them, no other tribes were threatened by the policy.

In 1961, when the New Frontier administration came to power, termination became a discredited policy. The new social programs of the Kennedy-Johnson years turned people's attentions to community development and away from the termination of the federal relationship. The Great Society programs of the Johnson administration opened up many developments for Indians. Community Action Programs were designed and operated by the tribes and they included everyone on the reservation, whites as well as Indians. While the poverty programs did not solve the problem of poverty on the reservations, they did give the people a chance to make many long-needed improvements in their communities.

One of the major factors in the development

of the contemporary Indian scene was the return of Indians to the reservations to work in the various tribal programs. Many Indians had gone to college during the sixties and after graduation they discovered plenty of opportunities awaiting them in tribal programs. The jobs were mostly administrative and this hampered some of the new graduates who had concentrated on liberal arts or education and who had little experience or training in administration. On the whole, however, the college graduates did a creditable job of helping the tribes develop and operate programs.

As the community-oriented programs continued, a process of re-tribalization began. The programs were designed to make maximum use of existing tribal traditions, but a great many of the Indians working in the programs did not know enough about their own heritage to relate to the community. The interest in traditions began to grow as people tried to adjust to the facts of tribal life. Ceremonies were well attended and not just by the traditional Indians. The newer generation made it a point to learn everything it could about the old tribal ways.

A serious generation gap began to emerge between the new educated generation and the tribal officials who had spent their lives on the reservations. Many of the tribal officials were very conservative and tended to protect what they had rather than try to get more for the tribe. This attitude antagonized the younger Indians, who became hostile toward the tribal govern-

ments. The relationship between the Bureau of
Indian Affairs and the tribal council dated back
to the days of the Indian Reorganization Act. Most
tribal officials refused to oppose Bureau policy
decisions because they appreciated the long-term
power that the bureaucrats exercised over tribal
developments.

The younger people refused to accept the
Bureau of Indian Affairs continuing to make the
decisions regarding the reservations. When they
pointed out the examples of corruption allowed
to exist on some reservations, they found themselves opposed by both the Bureau of Indian
Affairs and the tribal officials. In anger they turned
to the traditional leaders they had grown to
know during the ceremonials. Powerful coalitions
were formed on some reservations composed of
the younger, educated and more militant Indians and the older traditional people who had
never recognized the Indian Reorganization Act
governments.

During the week of the national elections in
the fall of 1972 militants of seven national Indian
organizations called for a march on Washington,
D.C. to highlight the conditions of Indians. In
this march, now known as the Trail of Broken
Treaties, they were joined by a great many reservation people. Eighty percent of the participants
were said to be reservation residents. The
marchers occupied the Bureau of Indian Affairs
headquarters and the government later claimed
that the occupation cost the taxpayers some 1.4

million dollars in damage to the buildings. A month later the National Congress of American Indians authorized a survey impact team to prepare a report on the damage. As part of the survey the staff asked numerous Indians if they agreed with the Twenty Points which the marchers had brought to Washington to present to the government. An astounding three-quarters of the Indians asked were highly favorable to the program suggested by the Trail of Broken Treaties participants.

It was this protest, not Alcatraz, that really set the Bureau of Indian Affairs on edge. After the participants had left the Bureau's buildings and people saw the damage caused by the occupation, many tribal leaders asked the government for special funds for more tribal and federal police to prevent similar occupations from occurring on the reservations. Only history will be able to tell if this move was proper. The additional police authorized harassed the political rivals of the current tribal chairman instead of protecting the reservations against an invasion.

At the Pine Ridge Reservation of the Oglala Sioux the tribal chairman was particularly worried about the American Indian Movement and its many followers. One of the leaders of A.I.M. was a tribal member, Russell Means, who had become a strong traditionalist follower and had participated in the Sun Dance for several years. Means had a large following on the reservation and was a political threat to the incumbent, Dick

Wilson. He was also a threat to the white store-owners and cattlepeople because he advocated cooperative buying techniques and the use of Indian lands by Indian cattlepeople.

Wilson's tribal police put more and more pressure on the traditional people, his political opponents, and on A.I.M. sympathizers causing complaints to Washington that the police were being misused and should be removed. The government did nothing because it was already committed to support Wilson's rule. Tensions increased while Wilson, safe at Pine Ridge, kept issuing taunts and threats to both the American Indian Movement and the traditional chiefs of the Oglalas. Finally, on February 27, 1973, two tribal police attacked Russell Means and his lawyer at the shopping center in Pine Ridge.

The next day a mixed crowd of protestors moved into Wounded Knee and occupied the tiny village. The rest is history. The occupation lasted seventy-two days and two Indians were killed, a federal marshal crippled, and thousands of dollars and thousands of people tied up in the confrontation. When the occupation ended the government did nothing to prevent further violence, and by the end of 1973, six Indians had been killed by persons unknown. The suspicion was that the tribal police had committed the killings, but with all the confusion and hatred on the reservation following the occupation, it was anybody's guess who killed them.

Wounded Knee seems to form a natural watershed in understanding the nature of current Indian problems. It is a climax of all of the confusion of the past century and involves the determination of the treaty issues, the land and leasing issues, the issue of Indian tribal religions and the issue of what constitutes, in 1974 and beyond, an Indian community. Some of these issues may never be resolved; others may become clearer and less emotional in years to come. Few Indians will forget that the Sioux and other tribes had reached a point where they were willing to kill each other to resolve these issues. Nor will they forget that the confrontation over the future direction of Indian Affairs occurred at that historic village where, on a snowy field, another phase of Indian existence ended in 1890.

4

Patterns of Resistance

It is very difficult to have lived through the recent experience at Wounded Knee and not to have taken sides at one point or another. The occupation seemed to polarize both Indians and whites to a degree not previously encountered. Many Indians were demanding, just as some whites were, that the government go in and clear out the village, even if it meant killing people. Other Indians and whites were solidly behind the occupation and wanted more occupations on other reservations.

The history of the Indian-white confrontation goes back to the days of Columbus and is characterized by frequent clashes. The European nations had no little trouble getting the tribes to follow their directives and even Great Britain trod a wary path when suggesting that their traditional allies, the Iroquois, embark on certain ventures. With the advent of the United States, much of the conflict between Americans and the Indian tribes was due to the inability of the American government to prevent its citizens from violating its pledges. No sooner was a land area promised to the tribe through a treaty than the squatters and landsharks would move into it and demand that the federal government purchase it from the tribe.

With the squatters and land speculators came an Indian dependence on the tools of the white man's technology. Fur traders and trappers introduced guns, steel knives, iron kettles, factory-made clothes and manufactured farm implements. The tribes became used to these new utensils and the people clamored for more trade goods. Conflicts broke out over trade and led to open warfare with the Indians coming out losers.

The traditional leadership of the tribes saw in this process a two-fold deterioration of the tribe. First, the tribe regarded the treaty as a sacred pledge of its honor and, when it found that the white people did not regard it as such, the Indians lost the whole basis of negotiations. They began to trust the United States less and less and began insisting on more specific wording in the treaties. When even these more specific treaties were violated, the tribe often turned to its traditions hoping that, by purifying themselves through their old ceremonies, they could restore the tribe to a place of primacy and strength.

Second, when the old traditions were reclaimed the people would find that a dependence upon the white people's manufactured goods had destroyed the confidence of the tribe to hold itself together. One factor seemed to emphasize and accelerate the other and many tribes found themselves unable to resist further intrusions on their lands and customs. Thus Indian resistance was always mixed with a religious or cultural revival in some way or another. The Cherokee resistance to removal from Georgia occurred at a time when Sequoia had invented an alphabet for the tribe and educational programs were transforming the Cherokee traditions into viable techniques for living.

In addition to religion, Indians depended upon the ordinary channels of change in their resistance. In 1831, when the state of Georgia attempted to enforce its laws in Cherokee country, the tribe filed an original action in the Supreme Court asking that its treaty be upheld. The court dodged the issues of the Cherokees' treaty rights and decided against them on the narrow basis that the Cherokee tribe did not have the right to file an action in the Supreme Court. A year later, when Samuel Worcestor took up the Cherokees' cause, the court reversed itself and upheld their treaty rights. It was following that victory that Andrew Jackson refused to uphold the court's decision and gave the orders to move the Cherokees to Oklahoma.

From 1846 until 1886 the Five Civilized Tribes made many attempts to get the United States to give their tribal governments some kind of official status within the Constitutional framework. In 1870 a report was issued by the Senate Indian Committee on the possibility of forming a special state from the lands of the Indian tribes in Indian Territory. Unfortunately the Senate concluded that the formation of an Indian state would violate the Indian treaties. The ironic twist to history is that the tribes eventually saw their treaties violated when the Congress merged Indian Territory and Oklahoma Territory to form the present state of Oklahoma.

In 1888, during the days of allotment, the Five Civilized Tribes held a conference at Fort Gibson in the Creek Nation. Delegates from twenty-two tribes attended the meeting and nearly three thousand Indians came as observers. Led by Pleasant Porter of the Creeks, the assembly drafted a plan of union of the tribes and agreed to submit the plan to the government for approval. The hope was that the tribes would be allowed to drop their formal and traditional government in favor of a new Indian-designed constitution. The government, seeing the plan for union go forward, acted to thwart the plan by demanding that the Creeks and Seminoles accept allotment immediately. In June, 1889, when the tribes were to meet again to formalize their agreement, Congress passed an act establishing the Jerome Commission and authorizing it to begin immediate negotiations with the respective tribes for allotment.

The same type of formal resistance could be

seen in other parts of the country. The Sioux tribes of the Northern Plains held out against all threats and bribes when asked to allot their lands. The government finally went ahead with the division of the Great Sioux Reservation in the summer of 1889, but the tribes began a systematic attack on the division with innumerable lawsuits concerning the manner of allotment. By the 1890s the various Sioux tribes were getting permission from the United States to sue in the Court of Claims for violation of their treaty rights. During the succeeding half century nearly thirty different suits were filed in an effort to get the United States to fulfill its obligations.

In the Pacific Northwest the tribes responded in similar manner to allotment. The Colvilles, while accepting the principle of allotment, petitioned the government to give the Indian allotments in one solid tract so that they could consolidate their lands in one section of the former reservation area. Their argument made sense. They declared that it would be easier to have all the tribal members in one place, making educational programs and other government services more efficient by geographical proximity. But the government policy for them was that whites and Indians should take alternating allotments in order that they live together as neighbors. A land ownership pattern was created, which served neither Indian nor white settler and the government refused to discuss any other manner of handling the affairs of the Indians.

The pattern of resistance clearly shows that the thrust toward solving problems has been a religious-political appeal to a sense of values expected of a society and that the appeal has generally fallen on deaf ears. As the twentieth century began the movement of resistance took on a national aspect and the subsequent movements of this century have fluctuated between resistance on the tribal or reservation level and sporadic efforts to organize the tribes on a national basis.

Perhaps the first movement of any note was that triggered by the Indian graduates of the government boarding schools in the years immediately prior to the First World War. For nearly half a century the government had been taking Indian children from their homes and placing them in government schools. As the generations passed through the government schools the students began to learn about other tribes who had previously been just a distant group of people to them. At Carlisle, Haskell, and other government schools a variety of tribal backgrounds could be found and as Sioux began to learn about Yakima, as Apaches worked and studied with Crows, and as other tribal peoples heard about the problems each tribe was having with the government, the Indian students began to understand that each tribe was subjected to irrational and casual dealings by the government. Even after they had graduated many of these students continued their school-days contacts and a group came together in Columbus, Ohio, in

April 1911 to plan the formation of a national Indian organization.

Following the discussion of the need for a national Indian group to articulate the Indian position and work for the betterment of the whole Indian race, a call was sent out to the Indian leadership around the nation to convene in Columbus in October of that year. Of the eighteen Indians planning the conference eleven were graduates of the government boarding schools and knew hundreds of Indians who they thought should be asked to attend. From this conference came the first national Indian organization, the Society of American Indians. It produced the first consistent national pattern of resistance by American Indians and lasted for some twenty years.

The Society of American Indians made little effort to involve traditional tribal leaders. Tribal governments were virtually non-existent and the only leadership in Indian country came from those who were educated and were working in their communities or in the federal government. Although the members of the Society knew that national unity was imperative if the reservation people were to survive, two issues destroyed the organization. The first involved the position of the organization on the Bureau of Indian Affairs. Some Indians wanted the Bureau abolished, while others wanted it reformed. Emotions flared over that topic and the fighting became so distasteful that many Indians withdrew from the Society.

The other issue that served to destroy the group was their position on native religions, especially regarding the Native American Church. Since the reservations had been established there had been an increasing use of peyote and certain mescal derivatives in ceremonies of the Native American Church by the traditional peoples of the plains and the Southwest. Many members of the Society of American Indians were Christians who regarded the use of peyote as undermining the efforts of the reservation missionaries. When some of the more militant members of the Society felt bound to support the traditionalists, the break came and the issue of traditional religion seemed to flounder. The distinctive religious beliefs of the tribes served only to emphasize what kept Indians apart. Perhaps the most important role of the Society of American Indians was its effort to instruct Indians in working together to change the United States' treatment of the tribes.

Following the demise of the Society, a number of national organizations tried to speak for American Indians. The National Council of American Indians was a notable successor during the 1930s and included many of the younger members of the Society of American Indians. The National Congress of American Indians, established in 1944, helped bring about the Indian Claims Commission and blunted the policy of termination in the 1950s. The National Indian Youth Council was organized in the early 1960s and articulated the demands of educated Indians.

In 1968 the American Indian Movement was organized in Minneapolis and St. Paul and by 1972 it had almost seventy local chapters. The importance of the American Indian Movement on contemporary Indian Affairs cannot be underestimated. It was the first national movement of Indians that came from the local communities and not from a group of established Indian leaders forming a national group for specific purposes. Local chapters of A.I.M. sprang up wherever Indians gathered to discuss their problems. Many of the positions taken by A.I.M. local chapters were progressive, even though the solutions offered did not always fit the problems.

From 1911 to 1973 Indian resistance was centered in national organizations and the determination of highly complicated and sophisticated issues. Membership in the Indian organizations was realistically restricted to those Indians who occupied leadership positions among their people or who had a sufficiently broad education to understand the complexity of the problems. With the protest at Wounded Knee, resistance came full circle. The religious dimension of Indian life, previously divisive and destructive in the national organizations, became the most important aspect of the occupation at Wounded Knee. Ceremonies were held almost daily and the negotiations with the government were carried on with dignity and with ceremonial preparations. The national issues of treaty rights seemed to become once again a matter of local concern.

We are now in that period of Indian history when radical and long-term changes are being made. No one can say for certain whether the trend of Indian resistance will continue to emphasize the traditional aspects of Indian culture and religion. Twenty-five thousand Indians are now in college and the professional ranks are being rapidly filled by knowledgeable Indians. As they begin to work on the many problems facing Indians there will be a return to modes of resistance developed in this century.

For some strange reason the more educated Indians become the more militant they are about preserving tribal traditions and customs. A whole new method of dealing with Indian problems seems to be emerging both at the local level and in the national organizations. We can guess the probable solutions to these problems, the coalitions that may be formed to raise the issues, and the complex inter-relationships which emerge as problems are solved. Most important is that we understand the long history of Indian resistance and the ways it has been voiced in the past. Then we can see that the current Indian movement is not really part of the recent American social movement, but only takes on temporarily some of the aspects of that movement. In a larger sense the Indian movement is a continuing resistance which has its basic roots in the Indian experiences of the last four centuries.

5
The Churches and Cultural Change

Many accusations have been made in recent years about the role of the Christian churches in Indian Affairs. This role goes back to the earliest contacts between whites and Indians and one of the first and most continuous contributions of the churches has been in education. Many of the earliest colleges and schools of this country were originally set up for the education of Indian children. Such schools as Dartmouth, Harvard and Oberlin were begun as Indian schools and gradually were transformed into private colleges.

The role of the churches in the education of Indians continued after the colonies broke with Great Britain and formed the United States. Many of the early treaties contained provisions giving the missionaries parcels of land in return for providing education. In the Ohio Valley and Great Lakes areas church groups received land for schools and by the 1830s much of the formal schooling of the eastern tribes was by missionaries.

One has to distinguish between the early missionary efforts and those of the later missionaries who came to the tribes in the West. In general the early missionaries were less inclined to become involved in the political affairs of the tribes and more concerned with providing good education and religious instruction. Many tribes favored specific denominations and often almost the whole tribe would become members. This was particularly true with the Five Civilized Tribes who strongly favored the Baptists and Methodists. A native clergy existed quite early among the Choctaws, Cherokees and Creeks and the social customs were simply transformed from older Indian meanings to newer Christian forms of gathering.

In the early 1830s four Nez Percé arrived at St. Louis asking about a sacred book they had heard about. They were referring, of course, to the Bible, and their arrival happened to coincide with a desire of many Christians in the East that missionaries be sent to the distant tribes. Instead of the more intimate relationship that had grown up naturally between the tribes and the individual missionaries, the new missionary activity took on the aspect of cultural imperialism and religious activities took secondary place to the involvement of the churches in the great policy questions of Indian Affairs.

From 1830 to 1871 the churches played an important role in the development of government policy in the field of Indian Affairs. Church officials served on treaty commissions as official members translators and secretaries and they often saw their role as helping subdue the Indians rather than impartially guaranteeing justice for the Indians. The result was great injustice to the tribes of the West, partly because the churches failed to carry out their promises in treaty negotiations.

One can easily compare the actions of the early missionaries with those of later years. The Rev. Samuel Worcestor, a missionary to the Cherokees from the American Board of Commissioners for Foreign Missions, played a vital role in Cherokee history. After Sequoia invented the Cherokee alphabet, Worcestor helped them get a printing press. Not only was the Bible printed in Cherokee, but also a newspaper, the *Cherokee Phoenix,* was printed on the press, indicating that Worcestor considered his duties to encompass all of Cherokee life. Worcestor and another missionary followed the Cherokee tribal laws and were thrown into prison by the Georgia state authorities for their loyalty to the Cherokee Nation. It was the Worcestor case that finally justified the Cherokee position.

Contrasting the role of Samuel Worcestor with that of other missionaries in later years, the difference is clear. Bishop Whipple, for example, and Bishop Hare, the Episcopal missionary leaders of Minnesota and South Dakota, were more concerned with the settlement of Minnesota and surrounding states than with the preservation of the

Sioux and Chippewa tribes. They played a very influential role in having the reservations of their states allotted. Bishop Hare viewed the change of government policy as a great arena in which to test the validity of the Christian doctrines. Commenting on the General Allotment Act, he noted that "Time will show whether the world or the Church will be more on the alert to take advantage of the occasion" (of allotment).

It was, of course, no contest, since the churches did very little to ensure that the "world" did not take advantage of the Indians. During the allotment process many church missionary societies were on hand to get choice parcels of land for their activities. On the Sioux reservations, for example, the churches did not simply get land for churches and cemeteries, but they also received choice grazing lands and used the income from these lands to support their own ventures.

On the West Coast the most famous Protestant missionary was Marcus Whitman. He had been sent to the tribes of eastern Oregon and western Idaho to provide religious instruction and education to the people of that area. He proved to be so intractable in his attitude toward the Indians that eventually they rebelled against him and killed him. In view of his intolerable attitude toward all things Indian, it is a wonder that he was not dispatched earlier.

Perhaps the most brutal of the church missionary efforts was that conducted by the Catholic missionaries in New Mexico, Arizona and

California. They saw Indians as serfs to be placed upon the lands of their missions to do their bidding. These people were not above waging war against the small Indian tribes of their region in order to convert them or kill them. The radical attitude of intolerance found in the Catholic Inquisition carried over in their policies toward American Indians until very recent times. As late as 1966 a Catholic priest was intruding into the lives of the Pueblo Indians by degrading their ceremonies and demanding an absolute obedience to his dictates.

The accusation most frequently made against the churches concerns the role they played in the passage of the General Allotment Act by Congress. Many church bodies saw the policy as a means of civilizing the tribes and sent a constant stream of resolutions to Washington in support of the Allotment policy. The Presbyterians in particular seemed to regard the policy as the special instrument of Christian activities in the last quarter of the nineteenth century. It was their opinion that as long as the tribes held their lands in common the Indians would be able to continue the old ceremonies and maintain the traditional community life derived from the tribal religions. On the other hand, the division of tribal lands would split the clans and make it easier to convert them as individuals.

The era of the Allotment policy remains a mystery to people today because so little has been written about it. Defenders of church policy have claimed that the pressures for division of tribal lands was so strong among the non-religious peoples in American society that allotment actually saved some land for the Indians. Until more research is done, it will be difficult to judge whether the churches were correct in supporting allotment or not. Bishop Hare expressed an attitude supporting allotment, but the churches then refused to get involved in the problems created by allotment and allowed "the world" to triumph over the Indians by default.

The educational role of the churches continued to be an important one after the establishment of the reservations. Although the government advocated the creation of special boarding schools, it was very slow in building these schools and the only education available to the tribes for a long period was in church schools. These schools taught a combination of American culture and Christianity which provided stability for the reservation communities. Many Indian community leaders during the 1920s and 1930s were trained in mission schools; without the church schooling it is doubtful whether many tribes could have maintained themselves as viable communities.

Resurgence of tribalism in the late 1920s and early 1930s stimulated the missionaries to oppose the Indian Reorganization Act and the Native American Church. Both the I.R.A. and the Native American Church offered opportunities for Indian communities to express themselves, but the missionaries did not see it that way. Many did

not appreciate the value of the indigenous religious activity represented by the practices of the
Native American Church and went to great
lengths to discredit those who participated in the
peyote rituals. The cry of religious freedom stirred
Congress to write guarantees of religious freedom into the Indian Reorganization Act to ensure
that the missionaries would leave the traditional
Indians alone.

An attitude of romance entered into missionary
activities sometime during the twentieth century
transforming the missionaries as this attitude en-
trenched itself. Earlier missionaries, while playing
policy-makers of Indian rights, had gradually become an important part of the lives of Indian
communities. The stories of incredible hardships
suffered by the missionaries in performing their
duties were not exaggerations. More than one missionary drove his team of horses through a bliz-
zard to minister to the sick and infirm and great
distances were covered by these people who
made themselves available to the reservation
people whenever they were needed.

In this century the missionary attitude seemed
to change. A missionary would come for a few
years, get a taste of the "white man's burden,"
and then move on. Missionaries became instant
experts after a few weeks in the field and made
no effort to understand the ancient traditions of
the people. Intolerance and impatience characterized this newer group and one of the first
tangible indications of this new attitude was the

refusal of the churches to recruit native clergy. From 1940 to 1960 many of the churches seemed to be deliberately avoiding the ordination of native clergy. Missionary work became a matter of expediency and not a mission at all.

The situation has changed somewhat since 1960 and has come to reflect what one can only call the "ideological" period of church involvement with American Indians. As the Civil Rights movement gained momentum church people began a subtle program to involve Indians in Civil Rights. Indians became, in their eyes, a sub-group of the black community; many lessons learned in working with American blacks were considered applicable to American Indians in spite of the cultural differences between the groups.

When the Civil Rights movement aborted and the "power movements" began, the churches abruptly switched their support to the more militant members of the Indian community. Much of the recent activism, both good and bad, was supported by church funds and given emphasis by church magazines and newsletters. Although not all of this support was bad, the attitudes which sparked such support were. Many high church officials were as intolerant of differences of opinion as their spiritual predecessors had been a century earlier in advocating allotment.

The situation is still badly out of balance. Many church officials, especially those at the national level, continue to deal almost exclusively with the activists and deliberately avoid con-

tact with the other segments of the Indian community. As a result, church funds for Indian work
go to support large demonstrations rather than to
assist Indians and whites in solving complex problems. Some of the churches gave funds to the
Alaska Natives to help them solve their land
claims problem; this money was well spent. But
when the Menominees sought financial support
to overturn their termination legislation, few
churches gave them support; instead they invested their funds in exotic and badly-conceived
projects of little worth.

Among the churches working with Indians one
group seems to stand out as more effective and
more concerned than the others. That group is
the Quakers. The American Friends Service Committee fought side by side with the Senecas to
preserve their reservation at Salamanca, New
York during the early 1960s. The battle was lost
and Kinzua Dam was built by the Army Corps of
Engineers, but no one can fault the Friends for
their work on behalf of the Senecas. They did
everything that a small group could have done.

In the Pacific Northwest the Friends have involved themselves in the fishing rights controversy. In 1967 they prepared a report, later issued
as a paperback book by the University of Washington Press, entitled *Uncommon Controversy*. It
is the best work to date on the nature and background of the fishing rights problem of the tribes
of Washington, Oregon and Idaho, even though it
focuses only on three small tribes. Fishing rights

in the Northwest is an ongoing problem charged with emotion but, with the exception of the Friends and Bishop Ivol Curtis of the Episcopal Church in Washington, few churches or church officials have supported the Indians.

One is always perplexed in attempting to evaluate the performance of the Christian churches in the field of Indian Affairs. National church bodies seem to be more concerned than the local or state church groups, but when policy is made by people two thousand miles away, mistakes are certain to be made. Such groups cannot be expected to be aware of all the developments taking place in remote parts of the nation. Yet church attention to Indian matters ebbs and flows. Not a single Christian church has a consistent policy concerning its role among American Indians. The Indian caucus has to do some tough lobbying at each church convention in order to save the programs for Indians. Every few years the policies of the churches shift, seeming to reflect the immediate concerns of the secular groups in American domestic politics, and Indians are expected to change with the new issues.

The commitment of the major denominations with Indian missions to develop a native clergy is, at best, weak. Over the last two decades one could only conclude that the churches will eventually give up all of their religious activities on the reservations. If this happens, the move may be viewed either as a final resolution of the Indian religious problem or as abandonment of the

Indians by the churches. For better or for worse, the Christian churches *do* represent a tangible expression of whatever sense of morality or integrity American society has left. As such, the Indian people need some clearly defined relationship to the churches, since the issues of treaties and education that must be raised with the government are essentially moral and ethical and require the assistance of the churches.

Appreciation of the long history of church involvement with the tribes is desperately needed. Some major Protestant denominations have a record of worth going back for centuries. Yet, with every new reorganization of the national church staffs, this history is lost or deliberately neglected by the incoming staff members. Misunderstandings result from dealing with church people who do not appreciate their own past achievements in the field of Indian affairs. Too often the fads of social movement are allowed to determine the course of action and continuity is lost. As the power movements gained popularity and the demand for the employment of minority group members escalated, the reorganizations of church national bodies simply eliminated many experienced people with significant achievements and experience in Indian Affairs in favor of temporary and token people who spoke the current jargon of change. This type of thoughtless disruption of relationships must be discontinued if the churches are to preserve any relationship with Indian communities in the future.

6

The Federal Government

Whenever people discuss Indian problems and solutions the great villain always turns out to be the United States government. The most popular accusation leveled against the United States is that it has broken every treaty signed with Indians. One cannot review the treaties without coming to the conclusion that the spirit of the treaties was never put into effect; if the letter was not violated, at least the spirit was and the treaties re-interpreted to mean something entirely different than that intended.

Treaty rights, so central to the solution of today's problems, have so many twists and turns as to make any statement on treaties appear to be an oversimplification. Perhaps we can best summarize the present situation by saying that the violation of the treaties resulted in the Indians not knowing their legal rights and responsibilities, and as time went by, these rights and responsibilities became so confused by both Indians and non-Indians that any solution became remote.

Let us take the 1868 Sioux treaty of Fort Laramie, which was the reason for the Wounded Knee protest, as an example. We can trace some of today's problems directly to the violation by the federal government of the provisions of this treaty. In Article I the United States promised that it would protect members of the tribe when they were away from their reservation. Yet there have been numerous instances where a Sioux Indian has been killed off the reservation and the federal government has refused to do anything about it. The question raised during the protest at Custer, South Dakota a few weeks prior to the occupation of Wounded Knee, was whether or not this provision of the treaty would be upheld by the federal government. Since the article had never been repealed, it seemed to the Indians that the federal government had a responsibility to protect them.

Article XII provides that no further cessions of land would be asked of the Sioux Nation without the express approval of three-fourths of the adult males of the tribe. Yet, eight years after the treaty was signed, the Black Hills area was taken from the tribe without their approval. The United States has not returned the land, nor has it paid for it. The Sioux are in a quandary. What did the treaty mean if they can get neither the land nor compensation for it?

What has happened is that the federal government has stalled for so many years that it now considers the treaty promises obsolete and nullified by time. When we look at the problems of other tribes or consider almost any aspect of Indian existence, we find the same situation. Violations have been allowed to continue for so long that the clearly articulated rights of Indians are regarded as nullified by the change of conditions. The federal government is the culprit, but in a peculiar way.

We immediately think of a three-headed monster when we speak of the federal government. This monster has a legislative, a judicial and an executive head and we must identify which head of the monster has failed to keep faith with American Indians. People in this century have tended to vest both emotion and belief in the office of the President and have failed to demand of Congress and of the courts the same degree of responsibility and concern that they expect of the President. The attention of both Indians and non-Indians seems to be fixed on the President as the person responsible for the conditions of Indians. This attitude among Indians may stem back to the days when the chiefs called him the "Great Father" in Washington and relied on his judgment in settling their disputes with each other and with the Bureau of Indian Affairs. With each new administration political pressure is exerted on the President to develop a program for Indians that will solve some of the problems. When the administration fails to deliver changes beneficial to Indians, the cry is raised: "The United States has broken its promises to Indians."

As one probes behind the scenes in the federal government, however, and begins to understand the political processes by which the government operates, the inclination to blame the President for federal failures appears to be an oversimplification of the problem. The Constitution clearly assigns to the Congress the major responsibility for Indian Affairs in two articles, the interstate commerce clause and the treaty-making powers clause. In the numerous lawsuits concerning Indians decided over the last two hundred years one finds that both policy and administration are clearly the responsibility of the Congress.

It is the Congress that must be blamed for the violation of treaties, since it was the Congress that passed the General Allotment Act, developed the termination policy, and has abdicated its responsibility for overseeing Indian programs. Almost from the establishment of the United States the Congress was involved in the determination of policies regarding Indians. It was not until the 1880s that Congress simply abandoned to the executive branch its role as policy-maker. At that time Congress began the practice of allowing the Secretary of the Interior to administer laws concerning Indians.

The Congress writes general legislation concerning Indians that it does not really understand, and to hide its misunderstanding, adds a clause stating that the Secretary of the Interior shall promulgate such rules and regulations "as are necessary to administer this act." This clause gives unlimited legislative authority to the executive branch, and although the legislation may clearly indicate an intent of Congress, the rules and regulations written to administer the act may very well promote goals contrary to what Congress had in mind. For example, in the Indian Claims Commission Act the government gave the Indian tribes the power and authority to sue the United States for past violations of treaties and for misuse of tribal funds in its role as trustee of tribal resources. These categories seemed to cover every cause of action which the tribes might have against the United States, but to be certain that the tribes had their day in court, the Congress created section five which allowed all:

> claims based upon fair and honorable dealings that are not recognized by any existing rule of law or equity.

The Indian Claims Commission Act was passed in 1946 after almost two decades of agitation by Indian tribes for a commission to settle treaty and accounting claims against the United States. A part of the pressure to create the claims commission was the persistence of two tribes, the Oglala Sioux and the Cheyenne-Arapahos, in seeking indemnity for the massacres at Sand Creek and Wounded Knee by the U.S. Army. The Cheyenne-Arapahos had been promised in the treaty of 1867 that the United States would compensate the families of the Indians killed or injured at Sand Creek, but the tribes had never been able to get compensation. The Oglala Sioux had a compensation bill for Wounded Knee introduced in Congress during several sessions, but each time they were opposed by spokesmen from the Army who maintained that the Wounded Knee massacre was actually a battle.

Congress included a clause in the Indian Claims Commission Act specifically allowing the tribes to sue the United States for depredations committed against them by the Army. The first claim filed under this section which fell into the depredations area was that of the Fort Sill Apaches. These people were descendants of Army scouts who had served the United States in the war against Geronimo. When Geronimo was captured and sent to a prison camp in Florida, the Apache scouts were loaded into box cars and sent with him. They protested that they were regular enlisted men in the United States Army, so the officer in charge told them not to complain and they would be reimbursed for their time.

The papers were never straightened out; of the seven hundred Apaches sent to the Florida prison camp, 670 were Apache Scouts and their families. A great many of them died in the humid Florida climate and the rest were shuffled around the federal prison camps of the Southeast until the late 1890s, when they were moved to Fort Sill, Oklahoma. In 1929 a Senate investigating committee visiting Oklahoma discovered their plight and again the Apaches were told that they would be reimbursed for their troubles.

The Fort Sill Apaches filed their claim in the Indian Claims Commission, but the commissioners decided that the tribe did not qualify for any compensation. Even though this section of the law contained no specific mention of land, the commissioners decided that the law should be interpreted "as if" the claims were restricted to land transactions. Thus, by a simple administrative declaration, a law designed to serve Indians and solve problems was turned into a law to deny Indians their day in court.

In 1920 the Congress passed the Snyder Act giving the Bureau of Indian Affairs permission to use federally appropriated funds to serve Indians living off the reservations. As time went by, the employees of the Bureau of Indian Affairs interpreted the provisions as permitting them to serve *only* Indians who lived on trust lands. At the present time the Bureau of Indian Affairs has many employees whose job it is to drive around the reservations checking whether or not Indians who receive federal services actually live on trust land. This practice applies particularly to those requesting college scholarships.

In 1934 the Congress passed the Indian Reorganization Act permitting reservation people to vote for tribal governments. Different regulations applied to the same reservation, depending upon whether the tribe voted to accept or reject the Reorganization Act. Under this act the Secretary of the Interior was authorized to return lands taken from the tribes earlier or to give to the tribes surplus federal lands located within the reservation boundaries. By the mid-sixties the Bureau of Indian Affairs had refused to follow this law and required tribes wanting lands restored to submit a bill in Congress through their Senator or Congressman.

We have seen a tribe wait as long as four years to receive a parcel of less than ten unused acres. The Bureau of Indian Affairs clearly has the power to return lands to Indians, but has stubbornly refused to follow the provisions of the law.

The Indian Reorganization Act also forbade clear cutting of timber on a reservation that had accepted the law. The Congressional reasoning behind this was that cutting of timber often destroyed the forests and left lands that could not be used again for nearly a century. The Congress wanted to ensure a sustained-yield program so that the reservation Indians would never be faced with thousands of acres of unproductive lands. The Bureau of Indian Affairs has continually violated this provision of the law claiming that it must get maximum financial return on the timber for the Indian people. Yet records show that the Bureau has consistently underestimated the amount of timber on the land and has used other practices to deprive Indians of at least 30 percent of their timber value.

One could give hundreds of other examples of how the Bureau of Indian Affairs and other government agencies have deprived Indians of their rights by refusing to administer the laws

properly or by deliberately changing the interpretation of the laws. People who understand this
process rightly place a major part of the blame on
the Bureau of Indian Affairs or the Department of
the Interior. Simply pointing out the nature of the
problem will not bring a change of heart and
mind in the employees of these two agencies.
Quite obviously, if these bureaucrats felt that
they were grossly violating the law, they would
make some corrections in their procedures.

The missing link in the whole process of providing services to American Indians by the federal
government is that Congress does not provide any
responsible overseer for Indian programs. It acts
only when forced to act, and then, only with
great reluctance. When Congress does pass a law,
it abdicates its legislative responsibility by allowing the Secretary of the Interior to interpret the
law. The only appeal to an administrative ruling is
through the administrative processes, so the Interior Department and Bureau of Indian Affairs
act as legislature, court and administrator of the
laws pertaining to Indians.

One might think the federal court system
would provide the balance that a three-headed
government is supposed to have, even if Congress
shirks its responsibility and the executive branch
is not responsive to the real needs of Indians.
In recent years a number of legal organizations
have been created to work in the field of Indian
law and the amount of litigation concerning Indian rights has drastically increased. Appeals to

the federal courts by tribes and individuals have achieved some remarkable gains, but we must look at the interpretation of laws to see how effective an appeal can ultimately be.

The federal courts must certainly be the busiest in the land. Recent Civil Rights and consumer protection laws, as well as the expanding number of ecological suits, have made the federal courts a favorite place to decide issues of general social importance. For this reason federal court judges must be generalists, and the infrequency of Indian cases in the federal courts generally means that the judges do not become familiar with the very technical doctrines governing Indians.

One of the doctrines of interpretation in the field of Indian law is: in the absence of a clear statement interpreting a statute or treaty, the courts will look to the administrative practices of the executive branch to determine how to decide the case. What this doctrine means is that, if a tribe signed a treaty with the United States and the Bureau of Indian Affairs or the Department of the Interior consistently disregarded the treaty for a period of years, the court will decide the treaty invalid; if it were valid, then quite obviously the Bureau of Indian Affairs would have respected and followed it.

It is not difficult to see how the federal government has deprived Indians of their rights once the Catch-22 logic of Indian law is unfolded. When the arbitrary actions of the Bureau of Indian Affairs are held to be the official position of the United States on the assumption that federal agencies follow laws and hence are the measure of what is legal, there is really no appeal for Indians except demonstrations such as Wounded Knee.

The breakdown in the federal responsibility is primarily a breakdown of the functions of the legislative branch, the Congress, when it abdicates its responsibility to legislate and to oversee. The tragedy of Indian Affairs is that Congress abdicates both functions to the lowest level of administrative power in the Bureau of Indian Affairs area and agency offices. The federal government has been derelict in its legal and moral duties to American Indians. Each branch of the government has failed in its task and tried to shift both blame and responsibility to other branches in what is essentially an unconstitutional transfer of powers.

7

Current Indian Problems

In this chapter we shall look at a variety of complicated problems requiring new laws or a different type of administration of existing laws. The problems are primarily legal growing out of the refusal by the federal government to clarify for itself and for Indians the exact nature of Indian rights and how they can exercise them. For instance, had the federal government fulfilled the educational provisions of the treaties decades ago, we would not have the current extreme confusion in education. Indian people are sometimes given conflicting interpretations of how they are to seek an education, indicating that one of our present tasks is to clarify the laws which govern Indians.

In addition to the conflict which has developed around the 1868 Sioux treaty and illustrated by the occupation at Wounded Knee in 1973, there are a great many other treaty violations which concern Indians today. Perhaps the most emotional and serious of all is the violation of the fishing rights clauses in the treaties signed with the tribes of the Pacific Northwest.

In 1854 and 1855 Isaac Stevens came to the West Coast to get the tribes of Washington and Oregon to sign treaties with the United States. Prior to Stevens' arrival, the tribes had relative freedom to trade with both the Americans, whom they called "Bostons," and with the British at Vancouver Island. The question of who owned the Oregon Territory had been settled in 1846 and Steven's mission was to place all the tribes on new reservations and open the territory to settlement. Through a series of six treaties he claimed to have gained the cession of most of the lands now comprising the states of Washington and Oregon. Whites poured into the territory over the famous Oregon Trail, beginning the rapid settlement of the Northwest.

The treaties were a mystery to the Indians west of the Cascades. Their religion told them that it was ridiculous to divide and sell the lands because the Creator had only allowed men to live on the lands and had not given exclusive ownership to any person or animal. They did not really care about the extensive lands in the area since they were primarily fisherpeople and were more concerned with the salmon and shellfish of the rivers and beaches than with the deep dark forests of the land. The Indians, therefore, had few objections when Stevens asked them to allow whites to settle the land, but they raised very serious objections to the use of the rivers and fishing sites because their whole lives revolved around fishing.

Because of the Indian objections, an article was inserted in each of the treaties guaranteeing the tribes the right to use their traditional fishing sites, even though the lands were to be owned by white settlers. Stevens enthusiastically remarked that the Indians, by fishing and providing food for the new territory, would be useful members of the new society he saw developing in the Northwest. The treaties had hardly been signed and the reservations established when the whites learned the commercial value of the fishing industry. At this time the salmon were so thick in the rivers that one could almost walk across on their backs. When a market for the fish developed the whites wanted it for themselves. A struggle for fishing rights began.

During the territorial period whites constantly harassed the Indians who attempted to use their traditional fishing sites and many simply abandoned fishing because of the brutality. The territorial courts generally ruled against the Indians and the federal government did little to protect them. When Washington became a state, the new government took an aggressive stand against Indian fishing. Ever since, the story of Indian rights in that state has been one of continual struggle to have the state government leave the Indian fisherpeople alone. Numerous cases have been taken to the United States Supreme Court and the court has always decided that the treaty rights are the law of the land. But the State Fish and Game Department absolutely refuses to abide by the court's decision.

In recent years the conflict has been reduced to a fight between three small tribes, the Nisqually, the Puyallup and the Muckleshoot, and the state of Washington. The state does not bother the larger tribes because they have the funds to hire lawyers and to carry their fight into the courts. The smaller tribes are very poor and have practically no legal talent available to them, so it is easy for the state to harass them. Other Indians have shown themselves to be able opponents of the state. Led by activist Hank Adams and the Bridges family at Frank's Landing, they have forced the state to back down on a number of occasions.

The Indians of the Pacific Northwest badly need financial and moral assistance; above all, they need an honest defense of their rights by the federal government. More often than not the Bureau of Indian Affairs and Department of Justice conspire with the state officials behind the scenes to deprive the Indians of their rights. Only the stubborn persistence of the Nisquallies has preserved the fishing rights for the tribes.

Another pressing Indian problem is the use by large corporations of the natural resources of their reservations. In some areas of the West, particularly the Rocky Mountain region, the tribes own some incredibly large soft coal deposits which have been eyed by the greedy energy companies. On the Navajo and Northern Cheyenne reservations Peabody Coal Company has gotten extensive leases for strip mining, beginning the extensive exploitation of both resources and people.

On both reservations the traditionalists have vigorously protested the leases, but the tribal councils went along with the Bureau of Indian Affairs when the Bureau recommended signing the leases. The problem is complicated by the influence of outsiders on the tribal councils while the reservation people, who will feel the effects of the mining, are kept uninformed until it is too late. In recent years ecology groups and traditionalists have protested and joined together to prevent the wholesale exploitation of the reservations. This caused some Indians to protest that the ecology and conservation groups are opposing tribal sovereignty. Tribal councils admit that their course of action may not be farsighted, but defend their actions as the necessary expression of self-government.

There is still no clear decision whether or not the Secretary of the Interior must obey the Environmental Protection Act when he authorizes the leasing of Indian lands. As long as this point remains confused, it will be impossible to compel the strip mining companies to institute reclamation practices. The mining companies have agreed to contract clauses requiring them to hire Indian employees wherever possible, but their fulfillment of such clauses is somewhat less than inspiring. One can only speculate on the extent of the disaster that will eventually be visited upon the Indian lands of the West by the strip miners.

In this dismal picture great credit should be given to the people of the Fort Berthhold Indian Reservation in North Dakota. Several years ago the Bureau of Indian Affairs and some of the energy companies put incredible pressure on the tribe to sign leases for the mining of their soft coal. They have very extensive deposits under their lands, but they are primarily cattlepeople and will need an undisturbed surface, if they are to continue ranching. The reservation people invited a group of Hopi traditionalists and a group of lawyers from the Native American Rights Fund to make a presentation on the effects of strip mining upon the land. They listened very carefully to both sides and decided that they would not allow strip mining of their coal. This action by the Three Affiliated Tribes showed that, if the Indians are given the facts and the right to make the final decision, they will generally make a wise choice.

The strip mining problem is closely related to the problems that Indians are having with their water rights. In the early days of settlement mining was the chief inducement of people coming West. Gold and later silver were discovered in remote areas, but without water, mining was impossible. This led mining companies to build aqueducts to transport their water supply for miles from rivers to the mines. The legal precedent developed, permitting water to be moved from river system to river system according to the whims of the first settlers in a region. Today the right to appropriate and use the water of a stream or river is as transferrable as any other kind of property.

When the reservations were set aside Congress intended that Indians should have the use of the waters arising on and passing through the Indian lands, but it did not always work out that way. As the West was settled and the government began massive reclamation projects, Indian water somehow found its way into the hands of non-Indian users. The most flagrant misuse of water occurred in connection with the construction of Coolidge Dam in eastern Arizona. The project was justified as a means of assisting the Pimas and Maricopas of the Gila River Indian Reservation develop farm land. Yet when the project was finished the political compromises made during the life of the project were revealed after its completion and the whites in the area ended up owning the use of the water. The Gila River reservation remained as dry as it had ever been.

In recent years the pressure for additional water has become extreme. New resort or retirement cities have been built in Arizona and New Mexico which require a great deal of water for swimming pools, golf courses and fountains. The only remaining undeveloped or unused water is Indian water and both the land developers and state governments have been very militant in gaining control of it. For years a provision in the annual appropriations bill for Indians banned the use of any federal funds for developing Indian water rights. The effect has been to delay for nearly half a century the development of Indian lands, only recently begun.

The water controversy today centers in three states: Arizona, New Mexico and Nevada. The Central Arizona Project, enacted into law during the tenure of Secretary of the Interior, Stewart Udall, threatens to take most of the water of the Navajo, Hopi, Hualapai and Colorado River Tribes for domestic and recreational use in the expanding urban area of Phoenix. In New Mexico the waters of the Rio Grande, which supply the Pueblo villages between Taos and Albuquerque, are being appropriated for use in the new development cities of that area. Over in Nevada water that should be used to keep Pyramid Lake alive is being sent out into the desert to the irrigation district at Fallon. The leakage during transmission into the desert is estimated at 66 percent and the marshes that have grown up in the desert from the water leakage are now considered more important than Pyramid Lake.

The Department of the Interior, charged by law with the proper administration of Indian resources, has always taken a curious position on the water for Pyramid Lake. For many years the department acted as if the law regarding Indian water did not exist and maintained that the Indians would have to prove some ownership in the water to use it. This stance was modified when the Paiutes at Pyramid Lake began to get national publicity and the Department of the Interior could no longer openly violate the laws of the land. An incident which best illustrates the Department of the Interior's stand on Indian water involves Walter Hickel shortly after he became Secretary of the Interior. On a visit Hickel talked with Ronald Reagan and Grant Sawyer, then Governors of California and Nevada respectively. Following their discussion Hickel announced that the only way to save the lake was to drain it! So much for the foresight and concern of the Interior officials.

8

Indian Education Today

One aspect of Indian life in which the churches have traditionally been interested is education. From the very earliest times churches have provided educational services to tribes and much of the money and energy devoted to the American Indian cause finds a natural channel in the field of education. Perhaps this interest reflects the great American belief that any group can be transformed into good citizens through education. In the past the federal government has so relied on education as to make it almost a magical elixir for the problems of all minority groups, but especially for those of Indians.

Indian education today is undergoing a total revolution in both concepts and operations. The old days of reading, writing and a smattering of arithmetic are gone. In their place are dramatic movements designed to break the endless cycle of educational problems faced by Indian communities. We shall deal with three aspects of Indian

education today, although it seems as if there are
a hundred important aspects of Indian education
that deserve our attention. We shall cover the
three areas most likely to have an impact on the
future of Indian people: higher education, Indian
culture and Indian control of educational institutions.

The most dramatic change in Indian education
has taken place in higher education, that is in
college and graduate education. For the better
part of a century Congress held very strongly to
the belief that "Indians were good with their
hands." Where the idea came from is anybody's
guess, but its effect was devastating. Funds for
Indian education were generally restricted to
primary grade day schools and sometimes included high schools. Some funds were put into
vocational education, but on the whole, academ-
ically oriented programs were considered far
beyond the scope and ability of Indians.

For the major part of this century the federal
government did not make available any college
scholarship funds for Indians; the churches can
be given almost all the credit for changing the
government's attitude toward higher education
for Indians. Almost from the beginning of the
churches' involvement with American Indians,
funds were set aside for Indian college scholarships. In this century the churches invested an expanding amount of funds in the college educa-
tions of selected Indians. The late Rev. Galen
Weaver of the United Church of Christ was the

pioneer in this field; the U.C.C. was the first church group to establish a scholarship fund for Indians and has provided leadership in this field ever since.

In time the other churches began scholarship funds for Indians. In 1960 the Episcopal Church and the United Church of Christ joined the Association of American Indian Affairs in forming the United Scholarship Service. By pooling their efforts the groups created an agency that could both put pressure on the federal government in the field of college education and give scholarships to deserving Indians and Mexican Americans. The U.S.S. proved to be a wise investment because the situation called for an outside agency to demonstrate to the government, especially to the Congress, that Indians could benefit from a college education.

College and graduate education began to open up to Indians during the 1960s because of the work of the United Scholarship Service. As more and more Indians received a college education, even more decided that they wanted to attend college. The movement is still too recent to understand completely, but the statistics demonstrate what a revolution has occurred. In 1960 there were fewer than four hundred Indians in college, the majority of whom were assisted by the United Scholarship Service, some had tribal loans and scholarships, and a very few had federal loans or grants. In 1974 we estimate that there are some 25,000 Indians in college and graduate school.

In 1967 the Ford Foundation and the Office of Economic Opportunity cooperated in establishing a program to help Indian college graduates enter law school. By the fall of 1968 nearly twenty Indians were attending law school. The Bureau of Indian Affairs, not wanting to be left out, found that it *could* fund Indians for graduate study. From that program a number of others was also justified in the fields of higher education, administration and medicine.

Community colleges have been established on a number of reservations so that Indians working for the tribe or the federal government can continue to study for advanced degrees. A Consortium on Higher Education has been established in Denver, Colorado to ensure that more and more opportunities are opened for Indians all over the country.

The second notable movement in Indian education today is that of Indian Studies programs. The early efforts in Indian education were designed to destroy tribal culture and traditions in the hope of solving problems by forcing Indians to conform to the white man's culture. In the last decade, as ethnic and racial groups have asserted the identity and traditions of their heritage, Indians have been in the forefront of the movement to preserve group identity. In the late 1960s several student protests involved the establishment of an Indian Studies program. The young Indians who occupied Alcatraz were students from the colleges and universities of the San Francisco Bay area who wanted to use the island for a cultural studies center.

By 1970 there were nearly sixty Indian Studies programs established in colleges and universities in the nation. The most important of these are at the University of Minnesota, the University of California at Los Angeles, the University of Arizona and Montana State University at Bozeman. These programs were integrated into the regular curriculum, providing extensive course offerings which attracted both Indians and non-Indians. A group of Indians and Chicanos established a college at Davis, California but the idea did not attract many other Indians.

Interest in Indian Studies did not only affect the large colleges and universities, but had great influence on the attitudes of Indians toward education. In the midwestern cities Indian groups formed what they called "survival schools" to teach their children about tribal traditions and customs. Tribal language courses were started in almost every important urban Indian center and interest in the old ways grew among Indians of every political persuasion, from activists to conservatives.

Community colleges on the reservations were seen as vehicles for preserving tribal traditions. The Navajo Community College and the colleges on the Sioux reservations all offered major courses in tribal culture and customs. Previously

people asked Indians how they expected to preserve their culture in a fast changing world. No
one ever seemed to have an answer to the question before the introduction of Indian Studies
programs. Now the question is not how to preserve tribal traditions, but whether or not enough
non-Indian culture and tradition will be taught in
the Indian schools to enable Indians to understand and live in white society.

The final important area in Indian education
today is "Indian control." The subject of Indian
control is not new, but recently received an im-
petus from Congress itself. In the post-Civil War
years the Five Civilized Tribes developed their
own school system and produced many well-edu-
cated people. During the days of Oklahoma state-
hood controversy the tribal school systems were
abolished by the federal government and merged
with the new state school system. It was a disaster for the Indians and they felt out of place in
the new schools. Illiteracy soared in the subsequent decades.

In 1969 the Senate authorized a Special Subcommittee on Indian Education, which ultimately recommended that control over local schools
be given to Indian people wherever possible. This
recommendation created considerable controversy. Millions of dollars were being appropriated
annually for Indian education and state school
districts, and the Bureau of Indian Affairs school
branch had worked out a very comfortable ar-
rangement to spend all of the money on pro-

grams of their own choosing. To suddenly find Congress recommending that these funds be placed under some form of Indian control created great consternation.

The recommendations of the Senate subcommittee were like a breath of fresh air to Indian people and very soon groups of Indians were demanding that Indian school boards be created for the federal schools and that contracts for the operation of schools be made with local reservation communities. Aside from the question of treaty rights, there has been no hotter topic on the reservations in recent years than Indian control of education. The Bureau of Indian Affairs has used every trick in the book to prevent Indians from having any voice in the education of their children. The education budget comprises nearly 60 percent of the whole budget for Indians and, the Bureau fears, if it is lost to Indian control then eventually all of the Bureau of Indian Affairs will come under the control of Indians.

The Bureau of Indian Affairs is correct in its fears. The demand of Indians for nearly a decade has been for "self-determination" which means that Indians want the deciding voice in whatever happens to them. Indian control of programs and policies in the schools and colleges is the test case for Indians. If the battle is won in this area, then the rest of the policy of self-determination can be realized.

As a result of this confrontation, every session

of Congress sees a number of proposals put forward that either advance or restrain Indian control of education. The Bureau of Indian Affairs is constantly refusing to assist local Indian communities in developing their own schools; Indians are fighting back in the Congressional hearings by pointing out the refusal of the Bureau to deal in good faith with them. So far Congress has generally sided with the Indians, but the task of turning the Bureau of Indian Affairs around and making it treat Indians as people is a massive one.

From this continual round of confrontations has come a number of organizations designed to carry the fight to the Bureau. The most important of these is the Coalition of Indian Controlled School Boards, also headquartered in Denver, Colorado. The C.I.C.S.B., or "The Coalition," is now working with over a hundred local Indian school boards in trying to take over the education of reservation and urban Indian children. The Coalition is the most efficient and sophisticated organization that Indian country has ever seen and is far more capable than the Indian political groups, such as the National Congress of American Indians or the National Tribal Chairmen's Association, in getting changes made.

In the winter of 1973 President Nixon impounded all funds for Indian education and refused to spend any monies for Indians. The officers of the Coalition met with officials from the Office of Education in an effort to get the funds released; they were told they would have to sue the President to make the money available. They did. When the smoke cleared, the President had delegated his authority to the Secretary of Health, Education and Welfare in order to avoid a precedent-setting decision against himself and finally he had to order the money released. The Coalition thus accomplished more for Indians in one lawsuit than the activists have by any of their celebrated events, for the monies went directly into Indian controlled school districts and allowed the reservation people to begin development of their educational institutions.

All of these movements in Indian education have contributed to the present positive aspects of Indian life. Of all the changes that we can foresee, the most important will be the day when the major reservations and communities control their own education. Indians are not far from this goal, and once achieved, the watershed will have been crossed and Indians will be on the path to total control over their lives. It is rather ironic that the federal government, which has been so efficient in destroying the political movements of Indian tribes attempting to have the treaties enforced, is falling victim to the simple request that Indians have some voice in their own education. It is almost as if the Trojan Horse of Indian control of education were simply waiting to be discovered.

9

What Can We do to Help?

There has been a residual feeling of sympathy for American Indians in every period of American existence. From Roger Williams to the missionaries to the recent outpouring of interest in things Indian, we have always been able to rely upon a portion of the American public to help us. In recent times the problem has been more one of setting priorities and clarifying issues than seeking support from non-Indians.

There are always financial problems. In education there are two very effective groups controlled by American Indians: the Coalition of Indian Controlled School Boards and the United Scholarship Service. Both of these organizations have excellent records and are not afraid to fight the power structure for what they believe is right. Each group has been willing to go to court to protect Indian rights; in this struggle they always need extra funds to hire lawyers, do research and carry the fight forward.

The American Indian Historical Society in San Francisco is a unique organization. It began with an effort to correct the poor image of American Indians found in textbooks and has since expanded its services. In 1970 and 1971 the Society sponsored the first and second conventions of American Indian scholars and brought together Indians working in the academic community to discuss the overriding issues of Indian life. In recent years the Society has sponsored extensive research into the question of Indian water rights. In late 1973 the Society's warehouse burned, destroying its whole inventory of Indian books. Part of the loss was covered by insurance, but many of the books could not be replaced without incurring many new expenses. We are hoping that the Society can quickly regain its momentum and any help given it will speed its rate of recovery.

Among church-related groups some do massive bulk mailing designed to wring the heartstrings of even the toughest person. Unfortunately, these groups often spend as much money mailing appeals for funds as they do helping Indians. Others spend a great deal of money on new buildings for their missions while their Indian parishioners still live in tarpaper shacks near the mission.

There are two church-related groups to which I always give something each year. One of these is Cook Christian Training School in Tempe, Arizona. Cook has a new program to help Indians train for the Christian ministry and to help others attend the nearby colleges in the Phoenix area for training in technical trades and skills. The other group is the St. Augustine's Indian Center in Chicago, the first church-related urban Indian center in the nation. It provides job counseling, family assistance and general activities for the Indian people of the Great Lakes area who are constantly moving into and out of the Chicago area. While other projects come and go, St. Augustine's seems to maintain a steady and reliable program for its Indian people. Both groups are controlled and operated by Indians.

As we have previously mentioned each major denomination has its own Indian program, and in general, these programs have been very beneficial. Most of them put funds at the disposal of the Indian advisory committee of the individual churches; they are always seeking funds to expand their programs of assistance to Indians across the nation. In addition to providing funds for Indian groups, these programs also provide information on the current state of Indian affairs. Some of them have extensive literature about Indians available.

Indian people have a great many legal problems, so there are a number of organizations in the field of legal rights. It seems that every new incident brings more people into the field of Indian legal rights. Defense funds are set up and special funds for other purposes seem to grow every time a new crisis arises. The problem with so many legal groups is that very few last long

and many of those that do last are not designed
to provide lasting changes. They are usually established to provide limited services to a select
number of people for their part in a certain incident.

Our greatest need in the field of legal rights is
to bring permanent solutions to very complex sit-
uations. Indian law is still in the formative stage
and many doctrines evolved over the years are
still not fully developed and accepted by the
state and federal courts as statements of Indian
rights. We need groups to do the extensive research and litigation that each complex legal
problem requires. The Native American Legal Defense and Educational Fund of Albuquerque,
New Mexico is beginning a large project in Oklahoma to assist both Indian tribes and individuals
in determining their rights. There is no more confused legal history than that of the Oklahoma
Indians and this project is designed to bring
them up to par with the other tribes.

The Institute for the Development of Indian
Law is in Washington, D.C. This organization
concentrates on the development of legal doctrines and background research into the nature
of legal problems across the country. The Institute
has published a series of treaty books for the
tribes of the nation. Not only are the ratified
treaties included, but the books also contain
unratified treaties and agreements made by the
United States with the tribes. Some of the docu-
ments have remained hidden from Indians for

decades. The Institute also publishes an education journal to keep Indians informed of changes in the law affecting Indian education. The Institute recently began to publish a Legislative Review to bring Indians information on legislation introduced in Congress which affects them.

More and more tribes are setting up their own special tax-exempt funds to help raise money for tribal development. The Lummi Indian tribe of Bellingham, Washington, for example, has a trust aptly named the "Lummi Indian Foundation Trust," or LIFT, which raises funds in small amounts for scholarships and research for its new aquaculture project. These funds are very important in helping local Indian communities assist themselves in developing the resources of their reservations.

A great deal more can be done than sending money and one of the most important is keeping Congress honest. Some of the most detrimental policies in Indian history have been put into effect because there were too few people interested in what Congress was doing to Indians. Today we have no Senators or Congressmen who are out to "get" Indians. In the past, when Senators Clinton Anderson of New Mexico and Pat McCarren of Nevada were in Congress, we had our hands full. Most Senators and Congressmen are very helpful to Indians, if they know that their constituents are watching them. Your job should be to keep track of how your Senator or Congressman votes on Indian issues.

In the old days we used to make sure that our friends knew who were the bad Senators and Congressmen. Today we list those Senators and Congressmen who are particularly helpful to Indian causes. In the Senate we have Senator James Abourezk of South Dakota, who heads the Indian Affairs Subcommittee. Senator Abourezk is perhaps the finest subcommittee chairman we have ever had. Other very helpful Senators are Ted Kennedy, Sam Ervin, George McGovern, Walter Mondale and John Tunney.

In the House of Representatives we have a number of outstanding Congressmen and Congresswomen who help us. Congresswoman Julia Butler Hansen of Washington has a long record of fighting for Indian causes; she once told a prominent Senator that she would run him out of the country if he abused the Indians in her district. Congressman Lloyd Meeds of Washington, who heads the House Indian Affairs Subcommittee, has an outstanding record on Indian Affairs and is highly respected by Indians all over the nation. Congressman James A. Haley of Florida has a long record of helping Indians and once stood alone in the House Interior Committee in his fight against the termination of the Colville Tribe of Washington.

With so many friends in Congress, why are the Indians concerned? We are now facing the most important years in Indian history in the Congress. In July 1973 Senator James Abourezk introduced Senate Joint Resolution Number 133, which would establish a two-year commission to investigate Indian Affairs and recommend legislation. A number of people scoffed at the Abourezk resolution, saying that it would be simply another study of Indians without any real effects. The text of the resolution, however, indicates that the commission would be the most important for Indians ever established. The commission would have the authority to hold hearings any place where there were pressing problems. It could study and analyze all treaties, statutes, agreements and executive orders of the government to determine exactly the rights of Indians. It could also study the policies, practices and structure of all federal agencies dealing with Indians.

It will be difficult to get this resolution passed and made into law. We already have had some indication that the Bureau of Indian Affairs and other agencies are afraid of what the commission might uncover. For the next several years, therefore, our task will be to get the resolution passed and signed and to support the studies that the commission undertakes. Everyone, Indian and non-Indian, can get involved in the work and progress of this commission to make it the most important ever established.

There is one final task. In spite of the favorable publicity Indians have received in recent years and in spite of the great interest shown by the American public in helping Indians, some advertising agencies continue to degrade Indians in their advertisements. Hollywood continues, in spite of Marlon Brando's refusal of the Oscar, to exploit Indians without any effort to correct the erroneous impressions of Indians created by the movies. There always seems to be people filled with prejudice and hatred who refuse human dignity to Indians and whose hatred continues to infest the land. It should be the task of anyone wishing to help Indians to remain alert to the injustices and abuses that exist in America. People should not be afraid to speak up and stand up against injustice. The condition of Indians will change for the better only if enough good people do the thousand little things necessary for a better society. That's all it takes to make a nation out of a conglomeration of individuals.